THE TRUE STORY OF A HUSBAND, BEST FRIEND, AND CAREGIVER

The Struggle Within

A.L. RANDLE

PAGE PUBLISHING, INC.
New York, NY

First originally published by Page Publishing, Inc. 2018

ISBN 978-1-64214-635-6 (Paperback)
ISBN 978-1-64214-636-3 (Digital)

Printed in the United States of America

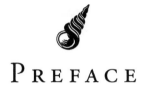

PREFACE

I wanted to start off by explaining a little about how I came to write this book. I tried to write this book during the end of my wife's treatment. As soon as I started putting pen to paper, two or three sentences into the book, my hand started shaking. I didn't understand what was going on, so I started writing again. My hands started shaking again, and then I started crying because all those emotions were still there from when my wife was first diagnosed. So I didn't write any more for about another two years.

When I wanted to try and write again, I kept making excuses to myself, my wife, and the publisher we had been talking to, that I didn't have time. The publisher called me one day, and I was upset and frustrated. I told them, "I'm not writing the book anymore. I am giving the book to my wife to finish, so you don't have to call me anymore." I wasn't frustrated at my wife or the publisher. I was frustrated at myself because I was searching for something, or something was searching for me. I didn't know what it was, but I knew it was close. I couldn't see it, but I could feel it somehow.

One day I was at work, and I was standing, looking at my surroundings, thinking to myself, *I can do better than this.* I wanted to be able to help people somehow. Then I spoke it out loud, "I CAN DO BETTER THAN THIS!" Not that my job was bad or anything. I just felt like I could do more or do something better. I just didn't know what.

The next day, my wife sent me a couple of articles. One was about this lady who was working three jobs and wrote a book. The second was about this gentleman that was a janitor that wrote a book while he was working. I called my wife and told her I read the articles. She told me, "If those people can make time to write a book, so can you." I told her she was right. I had no excuse whatsoever. I said to my wife, "Thank you so much for sending me those articles." Little did I know, my wife triggered something inside of me. I don't know if it was inspiration or what.

When I got off the phone with her, all I could think about was writing this book. I went to bed that night around 10:00 p.m. I woke up at 2:00 a.m. like I had been asleep for eight hours straight. Went downstairs and grabbed my computer bag. I plugged in my computer, opened it up. With no hesitation, no hands shaking, no emotional breakdown, I started typing faster than I had ever typed in my entire life. In three weeks, I had written fifty-six pages. I completed this book in less than two months.

It was around 3:36 a.m., the time I normally woke up from a cold sweat from my PTSD to go to the bathroom. That was normal for me those days. On the way back to the bed, I heard something like someone was crying. I put my hand on my wife's shoulder and gently rolled her over toward me. It was dark in the room, so I really couldn't see. So I moved my hand to where I thought her face was and felt wetness even before I made it to her face. I said, "Jess, are you awake?" She answered yes. I thought she just woke up from a bad dream or something. Even when my wife had bad dreams, I made sure I comforted her, and we talked about her bad dreams at that moment while it was fresh in her head. She told me she didn't have a bad dream as she was still crying. She told me her right side, right under her rib cage, was hurting really bad. Now I went into panic mode. Okay, let me tell you why. My wife has a little bitty voice, and she is about five feet, two inches of walking toughness. My wife does not complain about anything, and I mean anything. So like I said, I went into panic mode instantly.

I grabbed Jess and put her in our SUV. We drove to the nearest hospital emergency room, which was located on Durango Drive right off the 215 in Las Vegas. Once we made it there, I explained to the receptionist the type of pain my wife was in, and I also told her we had BlueCross insurance. I pulled out both of our insurance cards and gave them to her. I don't know to this day if it was the insurance or the painful look on my wife's face or the prayers I was saying up in my head on the way to the hospital, but they brought a wheelchair out to the waiting area and took my wife to the back in the blink of an eye. I think I got even more nervous than I was before.

All types of crazy thoughts ran through my head of what could have been wrong with her. I knew her backpack with her work computer was heavy, and I thought she might have strained a rib muscle or something. The nurse finally came out to get me and escorted me to Jess's exam room. When I walked in the room, she had this little smile on her face, so I thought that was a very good sign. Jess explained to me that the doctor had given her some pain medicine and an anti-inflammatory medicine as well. She said the doctor would be back after he looked over her scan. I was so nervous for that door to open to see the doctor. I felt like it wasn't going to be good news because the doctor was gone for so long.

Finally, the door opened, and it was the doctor by himself. He had this sad look on his face. He was trying to hide his emotions, but he couldn't. He looked like he wanted to cry. He told me and my wife that her liver was swollen from two cancer spots on her liver, and the pain she was feeling was her liver pressing against her rib cage. My wife's face went blank. Me, I had this big lump in my throat to where if I had started talking, tears would have started pouring. The doctor told us that my wife had stage 4 breast cancer. Right at that moment, my heart dropped. We both at the same time asked the doctor, "What does this mean?" We didn't have a clue about any stages of cancer except a lot of people that we knew, including some family members, had it, and they passed away from it. He explained to us about the different stages and said that my wife had the most severe, stage 4 cancer. I looked at Jess in disbelief, and she didn't know what to say. It was quiet in the room, and the silence felt like it lasted thirty minutes, but it was only seconds.

I asked the doctor if I could speak to him outside for a minute. I told Jess I would be right back. She said okay with her little soft voice. I walked outside, and the doctor had tears in his eyes. He told me he was sorry about the bad news he had to deliver to us and that his mom had passed away from breast cancer when he was a teenager in college. He told me he took his mom to all the different hospitals on the West Coast while he was going through medical school. He told me it was the hardest thing he ever had to do in his life. His mom started to see that it was taking a lot out of him for those three or four years she was around. He said that his mom told him one day that she was tired of fighting, and she wanted him to go out and live his own life. The doctor told me that after she said that, she passed away a few weeks later. I was doing my best not to cry because I still had that hard, sore feeling in my throat from the bad news he had just delivered to us.

What came next from the doctor was totally unexpected. It was like someone stepped in his body and took over because it was like I was talking to a different person. He told me, "Don't give up. Please do not give up on your wife. I was a kid, and I didn't know what I was doing. I was frustrated because I didn't have anyone to help me with my mom while I was in school." He said it took a lot out of him, but if he had it to do it all over again, he would have been more supportive of his mom and would have told her to not give up. The doctor told me, with tears running down his face, he would be right back to talk to me and Jess. He had to take care of some things on the computer concerning my wife.

I went back in the room, and Jess asked me if everything was okay. I told her everything was going to be okay. I really didn't know if everything was going to be okay. I was just trying to be strong for my beautiful little wife. I told her I had to go to the bathroom, which was right in her room. Luckily, it had an exhaust fan. I turned it on as soon as I closed the door. I started crying uncontrollably with my hands over my mouth. I felt like I had let her and her mom down in one big single moment, and it just all came crashing down on me in a blink of an eye.

You see, a year ago, my wife's mom passed away from brain cancer. I was the last person to talk to her on the phone before she passed away. I told her mom, Jean, that she did not have to worry about her daughter and that I would always be there to take care of her as long as I had breath in my body. Jean said, "Thank you, Anthony, and I love you." As soon as we hung up the phone, she passed way. My wife's cousin called me back right after we hung up and told me she passed away right after she hung the phone up. My wife was flying in from overseas, and I was going to pick her up at the airport in Maryland. I had to explain to my wife, once we arrived back at the hotel, that her mom had passed away. It was one of the hardest things in my life I had to do.

The more I thought about my wife not being around to love, hold, and to share my thoughts with, it made me feel like someone was pulling the love right out of my heart. I heard the door open to my wife's room over the vent fan while I was sitting on top of the toilet seat. I could hear the doctor asking my wife about me. I got up and wiped my face, flushed the toilet as if using it, and came out of the bathroom. My wife and the doctor gave me this look of concern, but they never said anything.

The doctor told us that if he sent us home that night, it would take a while to see a cancer specialist. The doctor told us that we needed to see one of the two women specialists in Las Vegas as soon as possible. So he admitted my wife to the hospital overnight, and one of the women cancer specialists would be in the next day to meet with us right away. They moved Jess up to the third floor, and I followed, carrying her clothes and handbag. I was so thankful that the doctor had gone completely out of his way to help us, because we were lost in this whole process and still in shock, to be honest.

Once we got into the room, I made sure that Jess was as comfortable as she could be. I knew she was tired because she didn't sleep that night from being in pain. Plus, the pain medicine was starting to take effect. Finally, she was sound asleep. As for me, I might have slept about an hour. The door was cracked open, and I could hear the nurses talking about my wife just being told she had stage 4 breast cancer. One nurse said she knew someone that had it, but they didn't make it. Then another nurse said that she knew someone that survived, but they had a hard time with the chemo. She also said their hair fell out, and they had to wear wigs until their hair started growing back. By that time, I was tired of listening to the nurses talk. I closed the door and sat beside my wife's bed and just looked at her until I fell asleep in the chair.

The next morning, I was hoping to wake up to a bad dream of us being in the emergency room. Nope, it really happened. I was trying to recall everything that the doctor had told me about the cancer specialist stopping by our room. I couldn't recall what time they were going to stop by. I told my wife after she finished breakfast, I was going to head home to take a shower and get her some clean clothes. I called our son, Anthony Jr., to let him know what happened because he realized Jess was not in the kitchen cooking breakfast like usual. Normally he would head to the kitchen and tell Jess about what happened at work or what was going on with him and his girlfriend. I asked him if he could come up to the hospital to keep his stepmom company for a little while.

Once he made it to the hospital, we explained to him what happened last night. I could see the tears building in his eyes as well, as we explained everything. I told him, "Everything is going to be okay, son." He asked me how I was holding up. I told him I was just really tired and needed to go get some rest. Jess looked at me and, with that little wife tone, told me to go home and get some rest. During that conversation, my wife's phone was ringing. It was her friend Abby from our neighborhood. Jess was supposed to go walking with her that morning. Abby knew something was wrong because my wife loved to go walking in the morning, especially with Abby. Jess was too tired from the morning pain medicine to talk and asked me to stop by Abby's house and explain everything.

I left the hospital around 11:00 a.m. I was sitting in my car on Durango Boulevard, right over the Highway 215. I was looking at how fast the traffic was flowing so I could merge on to the highway after I made a left-hand turn. Then it hit me, the wondering of my brain, the sadness of losing a loved one, my wife, my best friend. My thoughts were all over the place within seconds. My eyes were full of tears. I was gripping the steering wheel so tight you could hear the leather screeching. I put my head on the steering wheel, hoping all this pain and sadness would stop. The car behind me blew their horn for me to go. My eyes full of tears, I could barely see the turn or the line to stay in my lane. Normally, I was a sharp driver weaving in and out of traffic like I had lived in the city all my life, but that day, I was the worst driver on the road.

I managed to get on the highway, but everyone was passing me. I had the fastest car on the highway, and I was driving like Ms. Daisy. I finally got off at the next exit and managed to gather myself and wipe my eyes. I finally arrived at the front gate of our community. Once the gates opened, I just wanted to drive straight to the house. I made a right-hand turn to go to Abby and Alex's house, our neighbors and good friends. Once I pulled up to the front of the house, it took me a minute to get out. One, I was tired from not sleeping, and two, I was emotionally drained. With what little energy I had, I walked up their steep driveway, leaning forward with one hand on the leg that was leading every time I took a step to their front door.

My hand was approaching the doorbell when the door opened, and Abby had this concerned look on her face like she knew something bad had happened. She gave me a hug and asked me to come in to the living room. Alex went to the kitchen to get me some water. He came back to the living room and sat beside Abby as they braced themselves for whatever news I was about to deliver to them.

I started explaining everything that happened, from Jess crying, to taking her to the emergency room, to everything the doctor had said. The more I talked, the more Alex and Abby started to get upset. The more they got upset, the more I got upset. Finally, I told them I was exhausted and that I needed to go get some rest. Abby was a good friend and a very good friend to my wife, so I knew it was very hard for her to hear the news about Jess. They always went shopping and walking together. A lot of times they would cook together as well. My wife liked to call it girl time. I was so glad she had a friend like Abby, and I was sure Abby felt the same way about Jess.

Well, I finally made it to the house, and my two Old English bulldogs, Mia and Bear, came running out of my son's room. He forgot to put them in their room before he left to go to the hospital. Mia was looking around for Jess. When she couldn't find her, she was staring at me with her head turned sideways as if to say, "Where's Mommy?" Right then, I kneeled to the floor on one knee. She dropped her head and walked over to me. I put my hand on her head as she got closer and pulled her to me and gave her a big hug. I told her Mommy was going to be okay and that she would be home soon.

You see, Jess and Mia had this bond because Jess picked her out of this large litter of puppies. All the other puppies were attacking Mia because she was the runt of the litter, but Mia would always fight them back. Mia reminded Jess of herself. She was in gymnastics while going to high school. She was at practice a lot, so she didn't have time to have a social life at school. A lot of the girls were intimidated by her because she was built like a little bodybuilder. They always picked at her every chance they got, behind her back, but they wouldn't get to the point of wanting to fight her either.

Bear was like me, big, muscular, and loving, but if anyone messed with Mia or Jess, he would go instantly into attack mode. Well, Bear by this time wanted a snack. Mia wouldn't eat her snack because I think she knew something was going on. I put them in their room, took a shower, and went to bed. I didn't want to sleep too long, so I jumped up and set the alarm on my phone. While I was setting my alarm, you know how your brain has those flashbacks of the little moments that took place. Well, I was thinking about Mia. I was thinking how she would be walking around with Jess all over the house, and every time Jess would bend down, Mia would head straight for her chest, sniffing. She was sniffing like she was double-checking to see if her nose was working right, like oversniffing. I wondered if Mia had detected the cancer in my wife's body long before this moment.

When I finally woke up, after a two-hour nap, I felt better and could think clearly about what was going on. I was coming up with a game plan to help support my wife. I went on Amazon and started ordering cookbooks after doing some research about different foods to eat and what not to eat, like sugar, artificial sugars, canned foods, fast foods, etc. I was on a mission to help my wife after that power nap. After I ordered the nutritional books, I gave Mia and Bear a snack and promised them that Momma was going to be okay. Their tails started wagging, and they started running around, playing with their toys. I let them run around the house for a while, and then I put them in their room and drove back to the hospital.

It wasn't as bad driving this time. I think because I decided that I was going to do everything in my power to be there for my wife and support her in any way I could. Jess never gave up on me with anything, and I wasn't about to give up on her. The strangest thing happened when I was saying all this in the car to myself. Everything got brighter and brighter. It got so bright I had to put on my shades while I was driving. Once I made it to the hospital and up to Jess's room, she was up and moving around. She said the doctor couldn't make it, but someone else came in her place and explained everything to her and Anthony Jr.

I asked Jess, "Speaking of Anthony, where is he?"

She said, "I think he went downstairs to get some food." I was a little upset with him for leaving her there, but then I thought about it. My son could eat. He could eat a lot of food in a short amount of time. I said my thoughts out loud. "If he eats at the hospital, that's more food we have at home." My wife started laughing at the comment, which was a good sign she was in good spirits. Later, there was a knock at the door, and it was the doctor my wife said had stopped by earlier. He said he wanted to meet me and explain everything that he had explained earlier to my wife and son.

He started talking about getting Jess to chemo right away, and we could set up an appointment with the top breast surgeon in Las Vegas as well. He explained how many treatments she would need and how she would feel during the treatment process. He also explained about her hair falling out around the third or fourth treatment and that they had a place where she could buy wigs, hats, and scarves. He gave us a date and information on where her treatment was going to take place. Her treatment date was in two days, and her doctor was going to be Dr. Malata. My son walked in the room with a hand full of food and sat down in the corner, while Dr. Malata's assistant finished explaining everything about what to expect at our first visit to chemo.

After that, he asked me if I had any questions. I asked him if the place where we had to go was open today, and he said it was closed on the weekend. They try to get all the patients in during the week and have the weekend off. I told him that was the only question I had and that we would drive by the place on the way home. Looking over the directions, it wasn't too far from the hospital, which was good because we were already in the general area. My son told me he had to leave from the hospital to go to work and that he would see us later that night.

They wheeled Jess down to the front of the hospital, and she hopped out of the wheelchair ready to go. She was still feeling a little groggy from the medicine but was in good spirits for the most part. We decided to go home because she was missing Mia and Bear. We decided to drive over to Dr. Malata's office, at the chemo building, the next morning. Sunday mornings were normally quiet because people used Sunday as a recuperating day from partying so much on Thursday, Friday, and Saturday.

Once we got home, Mia and Bear knew right away something was wrong with Mommy because they didn't run full speed and charge Jess like they normally would. They walked up to her just wagging their little tails and placed their heads on each of her legs, as if to say, "We're glad you're home." Me, on the other hand, they charged me as to say, "We're hungry, where's our food!" Jess was going to get their food, but I told her, "No, just relax on the couch and I will get their food."

Once I got their food, I sat down with Jess, and we discussed about calling our boss at work to let him know we would not be returning to work anytime soon. We were working overseas and living overseas at the time, so we had furniture and clothes we had to get shipped back to the States. When we came home, we were on PTO (paid time off) for two weeks. So we had to coordinate a lot of moving parts, but we were ready.

Sunday morning, we drove over to the doctor's office just to get a feel of how long the drive would take. It was really easy to get there from the highway. Once we pulled up in front of the building, we looked around. It was just a plain brown brick building. It wasn't that big. I told Jess, "This place probably doesn't have a lot of patients like the hospital does. That's probably why it's so little." Man, was I completely wrong about that.

Monday morning, we stopped by Abby and Alex's before heading over for Jess's first chemo treatment. Abby told us if there was anything we needed to not hesitate to ask. We asked her and Alex to ask our prayer group to pray for us. She said she had already sent out an email to the prayer group the previous day I stopped by. We were so grateful for her and Alex for putting on such a strong face of encouragement for us. I knew it was hard for them as well. After talking to Abby and Alex for a while longer, I told Jess we better get going before traffic really got too heavy. So we left with Abby and Alex saying a prayer for us as we were walking out the door.

As we drove out the gate of our community, Jess looked over at me and smiled and asked if I was ready for all this. I said, "Yes, I am.

We're going to do this together." If I wasn't sure about anything in my life, I was sure about supporting her and being right by her side no matter what happened. I think my wife needed that answer from me at that time because that was one less thing she had to worry about. As we drove down the highway, we started talking about the places we would like to visit and go vacation at the most. Hawaii was our first pick, and the Fiji Islands were the next place we would like to visit. I told her once we get through with all the chemo and surgeries, we would find a way to go to Hawaii.

We had finally arrived at the doctor's office, which was shared with at least four other doctors and a chemo treatment area. When I tell you the parking lot was packed, it was so full that cars were driving up to the front door and dropping people off and leaving. I told Jess I was not going to drop her off and let her walk in the building by herself and then leave. I told her we would find a good parking spot, and it wasn't going to take long. Right after I said that, about two minutes later, we got a parking space right across the street facing the direction to leave. My wife thought that was pretty cool. When I spoke it, it happened.

We gathered Jess's favorite blanket, her computer, and some books. We walked in the building, and for a split second, it felt like everyone was staring at us. There were all different age groups, nationalities, men and women, but mostly a lot of women patients. The whole time I was thinking, while Jess and I waited in line to approach the counter, were these people here for cancer treatment or for something else? We walked up to the counter, and Jess gave the receptionist all the information they needed. The receptionist told us to have a seat and a nurse from Dr. Malata's area would be out shortly to take her to the back. I turned from the counter completely around and tried to scan for a seat as quickly as I could. People were getting up as their name was called, but also people were sitting down just as fast. We wanted to sit together as well, so I told Jess we would find two good seats, as we held hands. We finally found two seats side by side by the window.

Our wait time was probably about five minutes when they called Jess's name. My wife jumped up with no hesitation, ready to go. The nurse introduced herself as Maria and said she was one of Dr. Malata's nurses. Jess asked Maria if I could accompany her to the back of the office. Maria said, "Sure, everyone that comes here needs all the support they can get." I introduced myself, and away we went to the back, where the individual exam rooms were located. We stopped at the weight scale first, located by the nurse's station, to weigh Jess. They took everyone's weight that was going to start chemotherapy to make sure they were not losing a lot of weight while going through chemo treatment. Sometimes they had to make adjustments to people's chemotherapy regimen or dosage.

After Jess was weighed, Maria took us into one of the small exam rooms to take Jess's blood pressure. Of course, my wife's blood pressure was great. She was, as they say, cool as a cucumber. Me, I was a nervous wreck inside, and I was hoping no one could tell, but I was wrong. After Maria left the room, we heard someone at the door grabbing my wife's medical file from the door file holder. The door opened very quickly, and it was Dr. Malata. She introduced herself and went right into details about what was going to take place today. She explained to me and my wife that she had two large tumors on her liver that she was very concerned about, more than the lump in her breast. She told us she was very concerned because it could spread anywhere in the body once it got to the liver. Dr. Malata wanted to contain it to the liver and shrink it as well. Plus, she was going to give my wife some medicine to try and shrink the lump in her breast too.

So she told me and Jess that basically, she was going to give my wife a cocktail of chemo, the strongest chemo you could give a person. Dr. Malata's tone in her voice changed instantly as she leaned forward and grabbed my wife's hands and told her face-to-face. "I can mix all the drugs all different types of ways, but if you don't have the desire to live, then you won't live."

My wife told Dr. Malata with this stern look of determination on her face, "I am not going anywhere. I have too much to live for and a lot still left to do in this world. Plus, my husband and my son need me."

I think at that moment, or would like to believe, that my wife commanded her body in a way to start healing itself.

Dr. Malata told my wife about this lady that had the same determination as my wife did then, and it had been ten years since she had her last treatment and was cancer-free. I thought that was nice of Dr. Malata to share that with us, but I think my wife had made up her mind that she wasn't going anywhere. After we talked to Dr. Malata, she explained that Jess needed to get a port put in her chest first before they could start treatment. She said that there was a mix-up with the scheduling. One nurse had Jess in for chemo that day, and the other nurse scheduled her for a port placement after the chemo treatment. The port was placed in the chest, where the chemo entered and flowed throughout the body. They would place it on her left side because the lump in her breast was larger and located in her right breast. Dr. Malata told us that she would like for my wife to get her port put in place tomorrow and that she should not eat or drink anything after midnight.

The next morning, we decided to drive my GTR sports car over to the Henderson area of Las Vegas to the clinic. Jess loved riding in it. She was smiling the whole way down because I was weaving through traffic so fast. I wanted to make sure I got her there on time. Once we arrived in the parking lot, Jess told me that she had been nervous about getting the port placement, but the ride down in the GTR had made her feel better. I told her she could go inside to sign in while I found somewhere to park the car. She smiled, looked around, and said, "The whole parking lot has only three cars in it, and you're in a parking spot already."

I told her, laughing, "You know us men and our sports cars, we don't want anyone to hit our car, so we must strategically park." I gave her my big "Okay, it doesn't make sense to you, but it makes sense to me" smile. After Jess went in the building, I started calculating where would be the best spot to park my car. "Okay, I got it, over in the corner parking spaces but don't park it entirely straight." Once I parked, and after looking back about three or four times, I was good.

I finally made it in the building and found Jess sitting in the waiting area. They had two large waiting areas, so we sat in the left side waiting area. We were the only ones on that side. We sat there talking about the drive down and how hungry she was from not being able to eat breakfast this morning. I told her I would take her to go get any type of food she was craving after they put in her port. Jess's phone started vibrating, so she checked it, and it was Abby inviting us to come over tonight for Bible study group. We had not seen the group in some time, so we both were excited to see everyone.

About fifteen minutes went by, and one of the nurses from the back called my wife's name. Jess asked me to hold her purse, and when she gave me her purse, she softly rubbed my hand as to say, "I love you." It wasn't very long after she went to the back when she came back out front. I would say about thirty-five to forty-five minutes. I was like, "Wow, it felt like you just walked back there." She smiled and walked up to the front desk. The receptionist had just received a message from Dr. Malata's office to come in for chemo treatment in two days. The receptionist told us all doctors did that to give the incision time to heal.

We left and started driving to find Jess some food. I asked her how it was getting the incision put in her chest. She told me, "It was a male doctor and a male technician with a female nurse in the room. The doctor and the technician seemed a little nervous, because they were asking me how big you were because they saw us sitting together in the waiting room." She said they were nervous trying to make the incision for the port. I told her they had every right to be nervous. If something would have happened or went wrong, I would have been back there so fast it would have made their heads spin. I asked Jess if it was sore from the cut. She said, "A little, but not enough to stop me from eating a large salad, soup, and some fruit."

Later that night we went over to Abby and Alex's house for Bible study. Everyone was there, including all three Donnas, which always made it difficult for me at that time because I couldn't remember which Donna was which. Myself and Alex were the only men there that night with Abby, Jess, Donna V., Donna M., Donna G., and Nancy. After all the greetings, we all sat down, and everyone wanted to know everything that was going on with us and how we were holding up. Jess explained everything to the group, when we found out about the breast cancer up until she got her port put in today. There was a bunch of sad faces in the group after Jess finished, including Abby.

Abby excused herself and said she needed to go to the bathroom and she would be right back. She was gone for a good ten to fifteen minutes, but I think everyone knew why she left. Out of all the women in the room, Abby and Jess were the closest. Once Abby came back, we started our discussion for the night with the group. Afterward, we ended the study with a closing prayer. Everyone helped Abby and Alex clean the kitchen from the food she had prepared for the group.

I turned around and saw little Donna V. talking to Jess. When I say little, my wife was five feet, two inches and weighed 125 pounds; well, Donna V. was smaller than that. Donna V. always had a smile on her face and was always giving out hugs and sending prayers to anyone in need. After her and Jess finished talking, we left last after everyone else because we just lived right around the corner. We told Abby and Alex that we were going to be okay because we had our prayer warriors praying for us always.

Once we returned to the house, I told Jess to get ready for bed, and I would let the dogs out and clean up the kitchen. I was in, like, a supercaregiver mode or "superhusband take care of your wife because she really needs you" mode. I think she could see it as well because she was always giving me more kisses and tight hugs, especially when I was in the kitchen cooking. Jess would come up behind me and just hold me as tight as her little arms would let her squeeze me. When I had to move around in the kitchen, she would move with me, and we both would start laughing because she looked like a little football player trying to tackle a larger football player and holding on for dear life. Finally, I got everything taken care of with the dogs and the kitchen, and it was time for a shower and then bed.

When I walked in the bathroom, Jess had just gotten out of the shower and was towel-drying her hair. She asked me if I wanted to see where they put the port. I said yes. Once she showed it to me, I told her that it didn't look so bad. It looked weird but not gross or anything because it was literally right under her skin. It was small and round, about the size of a quarter with a rubbery nodule attached to it where they could put the needle into for her chemo. After she showed me the port, I took my shower and got in bed, and we talked a little more about what Donna V. told her after Bible study.

Jess said that Donna V. told her when she got her chemo bag to write on a sticky note, "God's healing love." Donna told her to always put this on her chemo bag and always say a prayer along with it. Donna V. did tell Jess she had been a nurse years ago, but she felt there was something else she was supposed to do, a higher calling for something else. Donna V. told my wife she was an energy guide, and she worked on aligning people's energy in their bodies. She suggested that we stop by her place to align Jess's energy before her first chemo session tomorrow. Jess was excited, so I asked her if she scheduled an appointment with Donna V. for tomorrow, and she told me she did.

The next morning, we got up and took Mia and Bear for an early morning walk around 4:00 a.m. There were still stars out. I told Jess when I was a kid and went over to my grandmother's house, which was a lot, by the way, she would always sit out on the porch at night and say a prayer while looking up at the stars in the night sky. My grandmother told me that anytime she said a prayer while the stars were out, her prayers would always get answered, sometimes fast and sometimes slow. I asked her, "Why don't all your prayers get answered fast?" She would look at me for a second, with those piercing dark-brown eyes and lines forming across her forehead, her nose flared open, with this look on her face like the all-knowing Wizard of Oz, "How dare you question me." It could have been I was catching her off guard, and she wasn't prepared to answer any questions, especially from her grandson. After that second-long pause and stare-down from her, she smiled and said, "It's God's timing, not our timing. Only he knows when it's time for us to receive our blessing from him." Of course, I acted like I understood everything she told me about the Bible, but I didn't. She would always make us read the Bible, and my brother and I never understood it.

I told Jess now that as the years went by, it all started to make sense. I told her that I believed that all your prayers did get answered when you were saying your prayers under the stars. I told her that was how we found each other. She asked me to explain it to her. I told her how I had just gotten out of a bad relationship when we both were in college. The person didn't love me as much as I had loved them, so we broke up. I was by myself for a couple of months. One night while I was walking to campus doing night security during the summer, I remembered what my grandmother had taught me years ago about saying your prayers under the stars at night.

Jess asked me, "What was the prayer?" I told her it was her. I asked for her, and God brought her to me. I asked God to bless me with someone whom I could love and who would love me just as much, someone who cared about me as much as I cared about them, someone who was very kind and loving. I told Jess I placed an order. She said, "Placed an order?" I told her, "Yes, placed an order." I told her I didn't know it at that time, but I figured if I was going to ask God for something, I needed to be more specific. I told Jess there were a lot of girls on campus, so I had to narrow it down. I asked God for an athletically built woman, about five feet, two or three inches with brown or blond hair, a nice voice and a cute laugh, and loved to exercise. My wife looked at me with this huge smile on her face and said, "You just described me!"

I said, "Exactly."

She was like, "Wow, that's amazing."

I told her the thing I had learned about asking for something was that you didn't ask out of desperation, fear, or greed. You had to be in a good state of mind, almost like a relaxing meditative-like state with good intention for yourself and for others. I told Jess, as we were on our third lap around our neighborhood, to say a prayer and be direct on what you want. She said a prayer for God to heal her body so she could be here to take care of me and Anthony Jr. And she asked that the two large cancer spots on her liver get smaller and go completely away. She asked that the lump in her right breast get smaller at the end of her treatment so the surgeons would be able to remove it. Jess asked for one last thing. She asked that if the cancer had reached her lymph nodes under her arm that it did not spread.

After her prayers, asking for what she wanted, she said, "Thank you, Lord." She was so happy after our walk. The dogs looked back at us to say, "Okay, we're done with walking. Let's go home." We took their leashes off, and they pretty much ran the rest of the way home. As soon as I walked in the house, I told Jess to go take a shower, and I would feed Mia and Bear. After I fed them, I made myself and Jess a good healthy breakfast with wheat toast, egg whites, organic cheese, tomatoes, spinach, organic sliced turkey meat, and organic honey for our toast. After we finished breakfast, I took Jess over to her appointment with Donna V. Once we made it there, Donna V. came out to greet us, took Jess right to the back, and started working on clearing my wife's energy fields. Donna told Jess while in the back room that her energy field was congested from stress, worrying, and toxins. She said that once she cleared them, Jess would feel a good sense of flow throughout her body.

When Jess came out of the back room, she was full of energy and was glowing with brightness all around her. Donna V. gave Jess a free bottle of immune-boosting essential oils along with some lavender essential oil for relaxation. We gave Donna V. a big hug and a good tip. Donna was still a student getting her license in aromatherapy and energy clearing and could not charge for her services until she was licensed. The money she took in tips helped pay for her classes and her trips to study with different energy level coaches around the United States.

The next day we had chemo. I say "we" because I was in this with my wife all the way from eating the foods that she ate, to doing the same exercises, to staying away from sugars, to going to the treatment sessions with her. This time when we went to the office, we found a parking space right under one of the shade trees. When we walked in the building, we didn't feel like newbies in the waiting area. We had this part of the routine down, with giving the receptionist Jess's info, to scouting out seats as soon as we walked in the door. We sat down, and yes, everyone was looking at us as though we didn't need to be there because we didn't have long, sad faces like everyone else that was sitting around us.

My wife and I decided, while driving over to the chemo medical center, that we were going to keep a positive attitude through this whole process. We knew we could do it because we had each other. We stood by each other for sixteen years for richer and for poorer, and now it was time for us to stand together in sickness and in health. We were not about to let that slip away over something like this.

Maria came out from the back and smiled at us both. I think she located us through the small glass window of the door, because we could see her as well. She called out Jess's name with a big smile. We both hopped up and greeted Maria with a big smile right back at her and asked her how her morning was going. She said it had been going really well that morning. Jess stepped up on the scale to get weighed. While Maria was adjusting the scale, she asked Jess if she got her port put in. Jess answered, "Yes, it was put in two days ago." Maria asked her how she was doing, and Jess responded, "I am doing great and feeling great." Maria then walked us over to one of the small waiting rooms to meet with Dr. Malata.

It was soon after we were in the room when Dr. Malata walked in with a big smile on her face. She told us that Jess had lost about four pounds since she last saw her, and she was just a little concerned with the weight loss occurring so fast. I went into panic mode again. I was trying to justify up in my head very quickly why Jess had lost four pounds in a couple of days. First my brain went into negative mode, and I could not control it. At least it felt that way. I started thinking, "Okay, we need to start chemo like right this second." Then my brain was thinking, "I can't lose my wife like this." I literally was crying, screaming, and on my knees on the floor in my head. I was hoping all this panic wasn't showing on my face, but it was, and Dr. Malata could tell. Her announcement of the weight loss triggered something inside of me.

Jess was very calm as she told Dr. Malata that we made a life-style change, not a diet, but a lifestyle change regarding our food. Dr. Malata had told Jess she could eat what she wanted. My wife told her that we had done some research and found that sugar fed the cancer cells. Also, she found that making healthier choices with food helped the body fight off the cancer cells, and the effects of the chemo were not so bad on the body. Dr. Malata said it might help depending on the person's body because everyone's body reacted differently to the chemo. Jess told her she was going to do what felt right to her body and that she would monitor her weight loss more closely because she didn't want to lose too much. Dr. Malata said that was her only concern. She didn't want my wife losing too much weight because a lot of patients lost a lot of weight when they first start chemo. She said some of them kept losing weight, so she would have to make adjustments in their medication.

Dr. Malata looked at me and asked me if I was okay. I told her, "Yes, I am okay," but she knew I wasn't. So she wrote a prescription for some medicine that would help me relax. I told her I didn't need it. She told me, "Yes, you do." I figured it was probably better to have some just in case than not have it at all. My wife agreed as well for her to write me a prescription. I guess by then they both could tell it was written all over my face. After we talked to Dr. Malata, she walked us over to the treatment area and introduced us to the head nurse for treatment.

It was a little overwhelming, to say the least. I was expecting something different. I didn't know what, but something a little nicer I guess. Don't get me wrong, the nurses were very nice. It felt like a lot of long faces, and no one was talking at all. There was music playing in the background for the patients, and they were passing out snacks in this little wood-like basket. The type you would probably see on a plane. Some of the patients said thank you, some didn't have the appetite to eat. Dr. Malata said goodbye for that day, while the nurse was trying to find Jess an open seat among the fifty or sixty brown leather recliners in this treatment area.

Jess turned around and told me it would be nice if we could get a window seat so we both could sit in a recliner side by side. The head nurse came back after finding us a spot over by the window. Jenny, the head nurse, told us there was an extra recliner right beside my wife's chair and that I could sit there. I told her, "Thank you, but I am going to sit in one of the visitor's chairs to the right of my wife." I told her it was a little crowded, so I wanted to make sure they had plenty of chairs available for incoming patients. Jenny smiled and said okay.

Jenny asked my wife what side they installed her port on, and Jess told her on the left side of her chest. As soon as my wife was trying to show the nurse where her port was, an older guy sitting across from my wife looked over as my wife pulled her shirt down a little to show the nurse the port area. Me, being the protective husband I was, started staring directly at him with this mean mug look. He looked right at me. I didn't blink. I was staring at him so sharply his head and eyes dropped to his own lap. He never looked back up at us even after he was done with his treatment.

My wife and Nurse Jenny were trying to find the soft part of the port. When the nurse finally found the soft spot, she told my wife she would feel a little pinch once she inserted the needle. My wife, the strong woman that she was, didn't feel a thing and asked the nurse how long she had been doing this type of work. Nurse Jenny said, "for about five or six years in the treatment center." My wife told her she was really good at inserting needles because she didn't feel a thing. Nurse Jenny asked my wife to say her full name and her date of birth while she made sure she had the right medicine for my wife. The nurse confirmed to my wife it was the right medicine and showed my wife the four bags, or cocktail, as we called it.

Before Jenny started hanging the bags on the IV pole, my wife asked her to put a sticky note on the first medicine bag. Jenny said, "Sure will." My wife wrote on a large sticky note "God's healing love," and below that she wrote, "Thank you." Jess gave the sticky note to Nurse Jenny. She paused for a minute, read the note, and gave Jess a big smile while she hung the first bag on the pole. Nurse Jenny hung the other three bags on the pole and said she would be right back. Jenny returned with the sticky note and some clear tape. She told Jess she didn't want the note to fall off the bag. At first when she walked off with the sticky note, we thought maybe we had offended her or something. We were happy to see that wasn't the case.

Nurse Jenny told us if we needed anything to let her know and that it would take about an hour for each bag and thirty minutes of observation after the fourth bag in case of any reaction to the meds. We asked her about the different bags, and she explained that the medicines were to shrink the two large spots on Jess's liver and to shrink the lump in her right breast. We wanted to make sure we knew what they were putting into my wife's body at all times. Jess and I believed that when someone was giving you or prescribing you medicine, you had every right to question it. At least that was the formula we had followed since we had been together.

As my wife started her treatment, I made sure she was as comfortable as possible. I covered her up in her blanket and made sure she had all her books and healthy snacks close-by. I checked her lines to make sure they were not hung up on anything. You know how sometimes you just have this funny feeling that someone is staring at you. Well, I had just finished checking my wife's lines that were going to her port when I turned around to see everyone was staring in our direction. At first it made me mad that everyone was staring, but then I realized something. Everyone in there was by themselves. I mean, out of the forty or so patients, my wife was the only patient that had someone in there to support her. As I scanned around some more, I noticed there were about three to four older gentlemen around the ages of fifty to late sixties, and the rest were all women. My wife, I later found out, was the second-youngest woman getting chemo in the room at thirty-eight. The youngest was twenty-six.

I was still scanning around just to see what else I noticed in the room with all the patients. I noticed the ones that did have appetites were eating a lot of fast foods, like burgers, french fries, fried chicken, pizza, chips, soda, and different types of candies. I could see all the boxes and bags from the different fast-food places. The smell was overwhelming because all that food in one area, and the combination was terrible. Luckily, we were sitting by the window, and it was open just enough to where a breeze came through to push the smell away from us.

Jess told me she was getting hungry, but not from smelling all the food. Her stomach was telling her it was time to eat. We started pulling all her food out of her lunch bag we had prepared the night before. Jess started off eating her chicken salad, which she made from a fully roasted organic chicken. We had also packed her some tomatoes, olives, and little, small cuts of beef sausage. For dessert, I cut her up some watermelon, oranges, apples, the core from the pineapple (a natural anti-inflammatory), seedless grapes, and two bananas. I know what you're thinking, that's a lot of food. It's not really. My wife really didn't eat a lot in one sitting, so whatever she had left over, I ate it. We have done that for sixteen years. I always ate what she had left over. I came from a family that didn't waste food. My wife told all her friends that I helped her keep her weight under control because I always ate her leftovers.

We finished lunch, and before we realized it, the nurse walked over to tell us that we finished the last medicine bag, which meant we had thirty more minutes left. During this time, I reminded my wife that she had an appointment with the breast surgeon on Monday. Jess was a little nervous about going, but she wanted to see what her options were going to be as far as whether having to remove her breast or being able to save it. Like I said before, my wife was a strong woman, but getting her breast removed or rebuilt was a little too much for her. I thought it would be a lot for any female, for that matter. Me, on the other hand, I didn't care as long as I had my beautiful little wife. That was all that mattered to me.

I could tell it was still lingering in her mind, so I asked her what she wanted to do after we left. She told me she wanted to go home and change so we could go to the park and play tennis.

I looked at her and said, "You're kidding, right?"

She said, "No, I am not kidding."

So of course, I was thinking she was going to get home, sit on the couch for a while, and then fall asleep for about two or three hours. Oh no, that didn't happen. She actually beat me getting dressed and was standing at the door with her hands on her hips, waiting for me.

All I could think about was kicking her butt at tennis. I was going to bring the pain as soon as we started the first game. We arrived at the park in the middle of the afternoon, and the park was empty along with the tennis court area. So I could really cut loose and clown Jess on the court. Me being the gentlemen I was, I let my wife serve first. Okay, that was a big mistake, a big no-no on my part. My wife served in her really unorthodox stance, so I just knew that ball was coming my way really slow. You know the type of ball that just barely made it over the net. I decided to stand flat-footed and yelled, "I HAVE THE SPEED OF A CHEETAH!" and that was when the ball flew past me. I didn't see anything. I heard the ball hit the fence behind me. So of course, I tried to play it off by telling her the wind was behind her when she served the ball. She said, "Yeah, that's what it was."

She smiled, but I didn't know how to take her smile because we were both in competition mode. This time I was ready. Okay, I thought I was ready. When she served the ball, it looked like it was in slow motion, and then it just all of a sudden went from slow to superfast and shot past me again. She was giggling and asked me if I was even trying to hit the ball. I told her I was trying, but I didn't think she was serving that hard. She told me she wasn't serving that hard, just her normal serve. I was like, "Normal serve my ass!"

She yelled, "What did you say!"

I said, "Nothing, dear."

By this time, I was down by two points. I didn't like being down by one point, especially to my wife, who's five feet, zero. So I did what I did best. I got mad and said to myself, "I am going to knock the crap out of this ball." This was my third mistake, by the way. She served the ball, and it looked like it was moving as slow as grass grew. I stepped to my right and swung my racket as hard as I could. I didn't care if I hit a home run out of the tennis court. My racket finally made contact with the ball! My hand felt like some electric shock went through it, and my elbow felt like it just got bent the wrong way. My hand opened up, and my racket went the same way the ball went—behind me on the ground, sliding into the fence. I screamed "Crap!" I didn't know whether to grab my hand or grab my forearm first. They both were hurting with the same amount of pain. My wife thought I just let go of my racket on purpose. I told her, "No, you hit the ball that hard." I told her I was all right, and we could keep playing. I really wasn't all right. I felt like I had just swung my racket into a brick wall because my hand was still throbbing, and my right elbow felt like it was hyperextended.

We finished the first game, and she royally kicked my butt. We played the second game. She kicked my butt. You see where I am going with this, and yes, she kicked my butt in the third game too. The whole time I was playing, I couldn't feel my racket because my hand was numb. I told Jess "You kicked butt today!" gave her a big hug, and told her she was awesome on the court. She gave me this big cute smile back, and I forgot all about my hand hurting.

That night when we went to bed, I could tell she was exhausted because she fell asleep before I did. Normally it was the other way around. My head would hit the pillow, and I would be asleep before Jess could even turn over to say, "I love you." I kissed her good night, and before I went to sleep, I tried to remember some of the healing prayers my grandmother had taught me when I was young. I couldn't remember any, so I put my hand on top of my wife's hand and said a prayer that I had been saying for years every night before I went to bed.

Now, what I am about to tell you, you can either believe it or not, but that night I think I was in between sleep and awake. You know when your dream is so real that you're emotional when you wake up from it. It was that real. You're awake, but everything is a little cloudy; you feel like you're floating instead of walking, and time is irrelevant. I remember praying for my wife's good health and healing. I also remember thinking about when I was little and had really bad migraines to the point I would throw up and start sweating so bad my clothes would be soaking wet. My grandmother always prayed over me. She would always put her hand on my head and close her eyes. I always felt a sense of peace when she did this, and I could feel the pressure leave my head. Then I would fall asleep for hours. The next day I would be running around like nothing happened. Like I said, it felt like time didn't exist.

I remember getting out of bed, my feet touched the ground, but I don't remember going to my wife's side of the bed. It felt like I floated over to her side. I was kneeling at my wife's side, and I remember putting my right hand on the exact location where her liver was. This all took place in the darkness of the early morning. I looked at my wife's face. I could see her so clear in the darkness of the room, and prayers just started pouring out of my mouth like water. My right hand started heating up. My left hand was hanging down beside me, inches from the ground. I do not remember getting up from the floor or getting back in bed.

I remember waking up to check the time on my phone. It was 2:25 a.m. I walked to the bathroom and turned the light on, looking in the mirror trying to figure out, was that a dream or was it real? I sat on the edge of the tub with my hands over my face, thinking, should I tell Jess about this in the morning or not? I got up and walked over to the sink to wash my face off. Looking at myself again before drying my face, I thought, *Wow, thank you, God, and thank you, Grandmother.* I was thanking God whether it was a dream or not because I believed there was healing involved with my wife. Dream or no dream, I was grateful. I was thankful for my grandmother, Retha, because she was always praying over her entire family no matter how good or bad they were.

That morning while in the kitchen, I asked my wife how was she feeling. She told me she was feeling great and ready to get the day started. I asked her if she remembered my hand being placed on her side. She said, "No, I was sound asleep." I asked her if she got warm at any point of the night. She said her body got warm like instantly but just stayed asleep because she though it was a reaction from the chemo. I told her I had kneeled down beside her and put my hand on her side, right over her liver, and prayers just started coming out of my mouth. "Really?" she said. I told her I didn't know if it was a dream or if it was real. It felt real until I floated, not walked, to her side of the bed. She said, "You were floating?"

I told her, "At least I felt like I was floating because of how quickly I made it to your side of the bed."

Jess's eyes were wide open with excitement and curiosity. She asked me if I could remember any of the prayers, but I couldn't. I could hear the prayers, and I assumed they were coming from me. It was like how my grandmother used to say her prayers. They just flowed, and she covered everything. Me, I was all over the place with my prayers. They would turn into a full conversation with God. Then I would forget what I was asking for. I would say, "I am sorry for not being able to say my prayers right." Then I ended my prayers with "I should have listened to my grandmother more when she prayed."

Jess said, "It's okay if you couldn't remember them because it was really early in the morning, and you did go back to sleep. So that probably played a part in you not remembering."

I replied, "Yeah, that's probably what happened, but I still can't determine whether it was real or not."

She told me not to worry about it and everything with her was going to be okay. We were meant to be together and grow old together. I loved the idea of that a lot and couldn't think of anyone else I would rather grow old with.

It was almost time for our appointment at the breast surgeon's office. My son was still sleeping because he worked at the dealership late that night. We put Mia and Bear in their room before we left. We got on the 215 highway that formed a C shape around Las Vegas. Once we arrived at the doctor's office, Jess went to the front desk to get her paperwork. The little reception area was full of women of all ages and nationalities. Some of them were so frail that they had someone helping them. Some were using a cane, a walker, or in a wheelchair. The majority of the women were by themselves. Myself and an older gentleman were the only males there. He looked over at me and smiled and nodded. I smiled back and returned the nod. He was with his wife, and they looked like they were in there middle sixties, were in good spirits, smiling and holding each other's hands. I wanted to tap Jess on her leg to say, "Look, there's a nice older couple, and they're holding hands."

I didn't want to interrupt her while she was filling out her paperwork. I was kind of glad Jess was completely focused on her paperwork because I didn't want her to look up and see a lot of these women thinking that she was going to end up frail with a walker or in a wheelchair. As a husband, I was just trying to take care of my wife's mental well-being. When she took her paperwork up to the front desk, she did glance at some of the frail women. I watched her facial expression as she looked at them. She had a sad look on her face when she sat down beside me. I asked her if she was okay. She said, "Yes. I just feel bad that there is no one to support them or help them." I told her I was thinking the same thing. I didn't want her to look at these women and think she was going to end up like them in a couple of months. I reassured her, "We have a plan about your nutrition, and I am going to do it with you." She grabbed both my hands and said with deep love, "Thank you, baby, thank you so much."

Before I could say anything back to her, the nurse called my wife's name, and we both got up at the same time, heading toward the door to the exam rooms in the back. The nurse introduced herself as Shawna. She walked us to the back and told us both they had received my wife's files from Dr. Malata's office. Dr. Melinda would discuss everything with us after she went over Jess's files. Shawna put us in one of the exam rooms and asked us if we needed any water. We told her if it wouldn't be a bother, that would be great. She said it wouldn't be a bother at all. A few minutes went by, and Shawna brought us some bottled water. She told my wife that she would have to put one of the patient gowns on for Dr. Melinda to check the lump in her breast, and she would be in to see us shortly.

A few more minutes went by before Dr. Melinda walked in, and you could tell she was going to get right down to business. She started off giving us some of her background, what she specialized in and how long she had been a surgeon. She asked us what we did for a living, and we told her we were DoD Contractors. I think she was trying to distract us with small talk while she was checking the lump on my wife's right breast. After she finished her examination, the small talk ended. She started by saying that the lump was very large and asked if my wife had started chemo yet. Jess told her, "Yes, I just finished my first chemo treatment, and I go again for my second session in a couple weeks."

Dr. Melinda asked how she was feeling during and after the chemo. My wife said happily, "I feel great!" We told her about the tennis match we had after her chemo session. Dr. Melinda started laughing when we told her how it ended with my hand being numb. Dr. Melinda said that was a good sign and suggested to keep doing what she was doing to keep her energy up. She also wanted to know how many treatments Dr. Malata recommended. We both said "Seven" at the same time. She informed us that the lump in my wife's breast would have to get smaller in order for her to do surgery and be able to have some tissue to work with to put an implant in her breast. Then she said something that neither my wife nor I wanted to hear. She said if the lump did not go down and they couldn't control the cancer in her breast and shrink the two large tumors on Jess's liver, then it would be probably best to remove both breasts. She also said they would have to remove my wife's lymph nodes under her right arm.

I am sure me and my wife both were thinking, "Wow, you started out taking us for a cruise down this nice street and then abruptly switched it over to a car wreck on the highway." Okay, I didn't know if my wife was feeling the same way, but that was what I felt like at that moment. Dr. Melinda told us she had to let us know about the different events that could take place, and she was not the type to try to hide anything from her patients. Despite that, I wish she would have kept that to herself because that did something to my man armor. My wife simply said, "Okay, thank you for giving us all the different options." Dr. Melinda said she would like to see us again after Jess's sixth chemo treatment.

The only thing that was going through my head was, *Well, I don't want to see you again, Ms. Negativity Doctor!* Okay, she wasn't negative, but she was just brutally honest. I mean raw honest, which I wasn't ready for at that moment. Jess had this poker face of a smile. I couldn't even tell if she was upset or not. She told the doctor thank you and that we would make the appointment on the way out. Dr. Melinda left the room, Jess got dressed, and we stopped at the front desk to make the appointment to come back after her sixth treatment. I didn't know about my wife, but I was ready to get out of that building altogether.

We walked out to the parking lot into the bright sun, holding each other's hand and not saying a word. We started the car up and got halfway down the road, and my wife's phone rang on the Bluetooth in the car. It was our boss, Lenny. He was calling to check on us and to get more information about what was going on. He was wanting to find out if we would be coming back to work or not coming back, needing more time to take care of things. My wife was answering his questions, and then he started asking me questions.

I couldn't hold it in anymore, and I just broke down crying on the phone. You know that man armor I was telling you about, well, Dr. Melinda cracked it just enough.

I was crying so hard I couldn't even talk. Jess explained everything to Lenny about what took place at the doctor's office. She explained to him a little too much for the both of us because then she started crying. Our boss got really quiet. I am sure he was upset because Lenny was never quiet. He was always joking, laughing, and clowning with people. If Lenny didn't talk to you, that meant he didn't like you and didn't want anything to do with you. That was the type of person he was, either all or nothing. After I was able to talk, Lenny told us both he would handle all the short-term and long-term paperwork for us and anything else we needed. We thanked him for everything, ended the call, and sat there on the side of the road for a while.

I told Jess I was sorry for breaking down the way I did. She said, "No, no, we both needed to let that out." She said it was probably building up in us both since the emergency room visit. I agreed, "Yes, it probably was, we just needed to let it out." After we wiped the tears from each other's eyes, I started driving again. We finally made it to the highway. The farther we got away from that building, the better we felt. Jess reminded me she had an appointment for a CAT scan tomorrow. I assured her, "I will take you over tomorrow."

The next day we drove over to the CAT scan facility right off Sahara Boulevard. It was a nice building, and there wasn't a lot of people there. We went in, and Jess headed toward the front desk. The receptionist told her that they tried to get in contact with her to let her know that our insurance said they would not pay for a CAT scan. Jess asked why they wouldn't pay for it. The receptionist told us a lot of insurance providers didn't pay for it because they did not see it as necessary exam. Jess asked her how much it would cost out of pocket, and she replied, "It's $2,000."

My wife said, "Really $2000.00?"

The receptionist repeated, "Yes, $2,000."

My wife asked the nurse if they took installment payments, and she said no, they could only take full payments.

My wife walked over to me and told me how much the scan was. I told Jess to sit down and I would take care of this. I asked the receptionist if they took debit cards. She informed me they could only take credit cards and cash, and no checks either. I asked the receptionist, "When they call my wife's name to go to the back to get her CAT scan, please let her continue with her appointment, and I will be right back with the money."

She assured me, "Mr. Randle, I will."

I said thank you and told Jess I would be right back. She was going to get her CAT scan today. She said "Okay, baby" with a big smile and gave me a kiss. I left to go to the bank to get the cash on Sahara.

You see, we had already done a budget for the year. I wasn't receiving a check from the company while I was off work with Jess; only she was, and it was disability pay. My wife was worried about where the money was going to come from. I knew she thought I had a secret stash somewhere, but I didn't. The only thing I had was a plan that I was hoping would work when I had to use it, but now wasn't the time to use it just yet. I got the money from the ATM and drove back to the CAT scan facility. I walked in, but I didn't see my wife in the waiting area. I asked the receptionist where had my wife gone. She said she went to the back for her CAT scan. I thanked her for trusting that I would be back. She said that she knew I would be back with the money when I asked her to let my wife continue with her appointment.

After I gave her the payment, I asked her what happened when a woman came in here and she couldn't afford to pay out of pocket. She told me they lost their appointment to someone else. I was like, "Really?"

She replied, "Yes, really, it's a business."

I told her I understood that, but what happened to the women that couldn't afford the CAT scan? She just shrugged her shoulders and smiled. I thanked her for answering my questions and walked away, surprised at how casual she was about the whole thing.

I decided to go for a drive around the surrounding neighborhoods while Jess was still getting her CAT scan. I drove up the street, looking at all the nice houses in the area. I made a complete circle and drove back to the CAT scan building and parked on the side to where I could see Jess when she came out. I sat there for about five minutes, and then all these negative thoughts started racing through my head uncontrollably. The thoughts came from out of nowhere, one after the other. I felt like I was losing myself in a sea of negativity. I was thinking about leaving my wife and just walking away. I couldn't believe I was thinking this way and told myself, *Okay, self, stop, this is not like you.* The more I tried to get it out of my head, the worse the "attacks" got. The voice said, "Leave your wife, I am trying to spare you the heartache of when she passes away, and she will pass away. You need to just leave her. You can't help her. You can't even help yourself. Just look at yourself. There are some weeks you can barely get through without thinking about killing yourself … days even."

I started fighting back by saying, "I may not be able to help myself some days, but I am going to help my wife get through this because I love her with all my heart. She wouldn't give up on me like this, and she's not going to give up on herself, so I am not going to give up on her." I started yelling, "Do you hear me! I am not giving up! Do you hear me! I am not giving up on her or myself for her!" Then the thoughts and voice stopped.

It was quiet in the car again. I didn't know what happened. It felt like I just got attacked, mentally. I didn't understand then, but I understand it now after hearing different stories about couples giving up on each other when one of them is faced with a life-threatening disease. They say that there is a 93 percent to 95 percent chance that couples will break up or divorce when the other is faced with a life-threatening disease. Well, at that time, I didn't know this, but it wouldn't have made a difference anyway because I wasn't going anywhere.

My phone rang. It was Jess asking, "Where are you?" I told her I was sitting in the car at the side of the building. I told her to stay inside, and I would drive around to pick her up. I had the AC on high because whatever I just went through in the car had me sweating and exhausted. I wiped my face off as best I could and drove to the front of the building to pick up Jess. She was all smiles and said that everyone was really nice. She told me to lean over to her, and she put her hands on my face and gave me a kiss. She asked me, "Why is your face so wet?" I told her I had the AC down too low I guess, and I just turned it up at the last minute when she called me.

That night we were sitting in the bed, and she was really quiet, too quiet almost, like something was wrong. I asked her if everything was okay. She told me that she was thinking about what Dr. Melinda had said about removing one of her breasts or both of them, and then she started crying. She asked me if I would still love her the same way if they took one or both of her breasts. I moved over closer and put my right arm around her waist, my left hand on the side of her head, and pulled her head to my chest. I told her I loved her with all my big heart, and we were in this together. She looked up at me with those big green watery eyes of hers and told me she loved me so very much.

We went to bed, but I think God had other plans for me that night. I fell asleep and wasn't dreaming about anything. I woke up around 2:00 or 2:30 a.m. to go to the bathroom, and then I climbed back in bed. I looked at Jess to make sure she was okay, and then I fell back to sleep. When I fell back to sleep, I started dreaming instantly.

I was at this funeral dressed in a black suit, and I was just standing there. I could hear everyone talking nasty about me. No one would come near me or around me like I had something wrong with me. I didn't know who was being buried. I looked at the size of the coffin, and then I raised my head. I saw my son standing on the other side of the coffin looking at me, just glaring at me, shaking his head. I knew what had happened then. It came to me in one big flash. Jess was going through treatment, and she was doing good. Her hair started falling out, and I got scared because I thought she was going to get worse. So I abandoned her when she needed me the most. Then I could see her lying in the hospital bed just before she passed away.

I woke up with this big scream, and I put my hand over my mouth, looking over at my wife. I got up and went in my closet and closed the door. God made me feel what my wife would have felt if I had left her up until her final breath on this earth. It was the worst feeling I had ever felt in my entire life. It was a very overwhelming sadness. A deep, deep lonely feeling of a broken heart, and out of everything she was feeling, she still loved me and was always thinking about me. I think that was what hurt me the most, that she still loved me after what I did to her.

The next morning, I was still in my closet. I put my ear to the door to make sure Jess was still asleep. I can honestly say this, when I walked out of my closet that morning, I was a different man. I felt an overwhelming love for my wife. Don't get me wrong, I loved my wife, but this love was ten times as strong as before I went to bed that night. I put my ear to the door of the closet again to see if I could hear Jess moving around in the bedroom. I still didn't hear anything, so I moved very quietly out of the closet, walked over to the sink to wash my face, and brushed my teeth.

As soon as I started washing my face, this little voice said, "Hey, what were you doing in the closet?" I jumped, and she started laughing. My wife was sitting on the toilet, watching me the whole time. I told her I had gotten up early to meditate and must have fallen asleep in the closet. I couldn't tell her about my dream, at least not right then. It was hard not telling her, believe me, because we always talked about everything. We made this promise to each other not to go to bed mad at each other and always discuss any bad dream we had the morning it occurred. So I told her I was clearing my thoughts to get ready for today and was going to do that more often. Actually, God straightened me out that night and made sure I was going to be there for my wife, like I promised I would. I can honestly say this: I was ready for any battle that came my way after that dream.

My wife even noticed a difference in me that morning. We went and had a good walk around the neighborhood with Mia and Bear. We sat down with my son, and he told us he was going into the army reserve and would be leaving for basic training in two to three weeks. He asked if we would be okay while he was gone, and we assured him we would be fine. That day I had to break the bad news to my wife that I had decided to sell my Nissan GTR. She asked me why. I told her I wanted to make sure that we didn't get overwhelmed with bills while she was going through chemo, and this would be money for anything that her insurance wouldn't cover. She said, "But I know how much you love your car ..."

I answered her, "I love you more, and it is just a car." Plus, I had already talked to the dealership about buying it from me.

I sold it for way more because they thought I said on the phone that the mileage was 35,000 and when I arrived at the dealership, they wanted to take it out on a test drive. When they got in the car, it took them forever to leave. I thought something was wrong. The two dealership guys got out of the car and walked straight over to me and said, "Hey, I thought you said it had 35,000 miles on it."

I replied, "No, I said it had 3,500 miles on it, not 35,000."

They told me it was still a brand-new car, and they didn't need to test drive it as far as they were concerned. I left there with a good-sized check, enough to cover a lot of the bills that were already piling up in a short amount of time.

Before we knew it, it was time for Jess's second chemo treatment. We went into the treatment building, but this time we went in like seasoned veterans. Jess went to the front desk while I found us some good seats close to the TV and near the nurses' door to Dr. Malata's area. Jess came over, sat down, and told me she had to start doing blood work every time she came in for treatment. She told me it was for Dr. Malata to keep track of her white and red blood cell counts. Right after she told me this, they called her name, and she walked to the door on the opposite side of the waiting area.

It only took them about ten or fifteen minutes to draw blood, and Jess was back out in the waiting room with me. We talked about the different healthy foods we could make for dinner that night and what we were going to do after her chemo session today. I told her I thought it would be nice if we went to the movies after we left chemo treatment today. She was excited because she loved going to the movies and catching a matinee. It was Thursday, which meant everyone was at work, and the theater would be empty. We talked a little bit more, and a different nurse came to the door this time and called out my wife's name.

The nurse's name was Rachel. She was really nice and very polite. She weighed Jess in. She had lost about three pounds from the walking and playing tennis for the last two or three weeks. As you can tell, I was a little more in tuned this time than I was the last time. Nurse Rachel took us into one of the exam rooms and checked Jess's blood pressure, which was good by the way. Rachel asked her how she was doing, and she said she felt really good. The nurse asked Jess if she got sick after the first chemo treatment. My wife answered happily, "No, I did not." She said that she didn't have to take the antinausea medicine the doctor gave her either. The nurse said that was great. She had to give Jess a white cell booster shot because her white cell count had dropped a little. Dr. Malata checked her blood work that morning and said that Jess's white cell count was good, but she thought they could be a little better than what they were, especially if she had chemo treatment that day.

The nurse gave Jess her shot, and soon after, Dr. Malata walked in the room. She had this big smile on her face. She told Jess she was doing great, and her body was responding very well to the chemo cocktail. She said that the white cell booster shot was precautionary because she had chemo today. That was one thing about Dr. Malata; no matter what she had going on in her life, she always tried to walk through that door with a smile on her face.

Dr. Malata wanted to check the lump on Jess's breast to make sure it wasn't getting any larger. After she checked, she said it still felt the same size and that it was very rare that it would start shrinking after the first treatment. Jess got dressed, and we told Dr. Malata how grateful we were for her and to have her as our doctor. I think she needed to hear that right then because she said she had a hard time with a patient right before our appointment, and it took a lot out of her. She said she was always glad to see us no matter how her day was going. We told her we didn't want to take up too much of her time because we knew she had a long day ahead of her. She put her hand in the air as if to say they could wait. She smiled as she gave Jess a big hug.

We headed over to the chemo area, walked in, and noticed there wasn't a lot of people there this time. We asked one of the nurses about all the open seats. She said a lot of people came in early as soon as the doors opened. Hey, we were not complaining, because we could pick any seat we wanted. We went over to the left side by the window, our favorite sitting area. I did my routine by making sure Jess was comfortable. I got her computer out while the nurse was setting Jess up with the big chemo bags first. The nurse went through checking Jess's tube to make sure there was no air in her lines from her chest to the bag. I set up Jess's computer for her and pulled out her cookbooks. I covered her up with her blankets because I could tell she was cold.

I told her if she wanted to, she could sleep, and I would be here to watch over here. She said okay and fell asleep instantly with a smile on her face. I was sitting there, smiling, just looking at her. I was thinking, *I wish I could take her to a beach somewhere or take her to Hawaii.* The beach was her favorite place. I thought about it helping her to heal by being in a relaxed area other than at home. It was relaxing at home, but I knew how much she loved the beach. Hawaii would be great because we could fly right out of Las Vegas to LAX or Seattle, Washington, straight to Hawaii. *That would be so cool,* I thought to myself. I sat there and prayed about it for a while still looking at my little beautiful wife all balled up in the recliner.

After a while, the nurse came over to change out Jess's last chemo bag. Jess woke up and was instantly hungry. We just had thirty minutes to go when I realized Jess hadn't eaten anything. I told her I would be back with a surprise for her. I went to one of her favorite food places in Vegas and got her a tomato bisque soup, a grilled turkey sandwich, cob salad, and a small bowl of fruit. The food was fresh, and they made it right there in front of you. It was always a crowd of people standing in line during lunchtime. I think she knew what I was bringing her back. We knew each other that well.

When I made it back, she could smell the food especially her favorite tomato bisque soup. She was eating so fast I had to slow her down, but it was a good thing she had an appetite. Usually she would have to slow me down from eating so fast. A few minutes after we finished eating, the buzzer went off in the machine, and it was time to go. We left and drove straight to the movie theater.

The third treatment went relatively the same way, and Jess's white cell numbers on her blood work were good, so she didn't have to get another white cell booster shot. Around the fourth treatment and the fifth treatment, the tumors on her liver started to shrink down to half the size they were. We were so happy to hear the good news from Dr. Malata. She said for some reason it took till the fourth treatment for everything to start showing some type of change. I was sitting there, saying, "Thank you, God, and thank you, Jesus! Thank you both so very much!" I was thanking them both for keeping us together, for keeping Jess's body strong through her treatment, for showing that love, hope, and prayers can get you through anything.

Even though we still had three more treatments to go, we knew everything was going to be okay with my wife's healing. We both thanked Dr. Malata because she told us from the beginning, "If you want to live, you will live." We thanked her for being honest that day when we first met.

My wife was on her sixth treatment. That morning we went in early. There wasn't anything out of the ordinary going on that day. It was just treatment as usual when we went into the treatment room after we talked to Dr. Malata. By the way, she confirmed that the tumors on my wife's liver and the lump in my wife's breast were still shrinking. Before my wife started doing chemo, the tumors on her liver were so large that it was causing her liver to hit her rib cage, causing her severe pain. Jess had to take anti-inflammatories a lot to reduce the swelling, so you can understand why we were so happy.

We entered the treatment area, and *wow*, it was packed full of people. All the chairs were full. I think they had about sixty chairs, and all of them were filled except over to the right side. We always liked sitting to the left because it was less drama in the seats on the left side of the room. It seemed like all the noisy, loud people sat on the right side back by the window.

The nurse pointed to the right and told us to follow her. Up in my head, I yelled, Crap! *I really don't want to sit over here.* But we were heading that direction anyway. Once we were in that area, everyone started staring at us like we were from another planet. My wife felt really uncomfortable over there because all the women were staring at her. I reassured her, "Don't worry about them and just relax. I am here, baby." She relaxed a little bit. This one lady was really locked on my wife for some reason, so I was staring at her to get her to stop staring at my wife. Finally, she stopped.

When the nurse arrived to put the needle in the woman's port, she started flipping out, threw herself out of her chair, and screamed at the top of her lungs while lying on the floor, kicking. She screamed, "I CAN'T DO THIS ANYMORE. I JUST WANT TO GIVE UP. I CAN'T DO THIS ANYMORE. I CAN'T DO THIS BY MYSELF. I JUST WANT TO GIVE UP. I'M IN SO MUCH PAIN, SO MUCH PAIN." The nurse was trying to restrain her from hurting herself. Finally, they had to give her something to relax her. Then they got her back into her chair. Whatever they gave her was very quick acting. The nurses were finally able to get to her port so she could reinstall the needle back into her chest. She looked over at me and my wife and then dropped her head and closed her eyes.

At that moment, I came to the realization that everyone needed some type of support no matter what they were going through, medical condition or not. It made me very thankful that God let me see ahead what would have happened if I had walked away from Jess. I grabbed my wife's hand, leaned over, and told her that I loved her very much. She gave me this beautiful big smile and sweetly said, "I love you too, and I am so glad you're here with me." Before we knew it, everyone started leaving one at a time. The right side was clearing out faster than the left side of the room. The lady that was screaming left and apologized to the nurse as she walked out of the chemo area.

We left soon after she did, and we discussed on the way home what had happened to that woman and why she broke down the way she did. My wife said, "See, you wonder why I am always hugging on you and grabbing your hand to hold and saying I love you about twenty or thirty times a day … because we are each other's support. When I am down or sick, you support me, and when you are down or sick, I support you." She continued, "See, we make a great team."

I replied, "Yes, we do, baby. Yes, we do."

The following Monday, Jess had an appointment to see Dr. Melinda again. We had a good relaxing weekend going into Monday, and we had some good news as well about the tumors shrinking. So going to see Dr. Melinda was completely different this time, even if she was brutally honest last time. We walked into the waiting area, and there was only about three or four people in the waiting area this time. It was not like the first time, where the line was out the door.

The nurse came out and took us to the back and asked how we were doing. We both said, "We are doing good, how about you?" She told us she was doing okay as well and said to Jess, "Mrs. Randle you look really good today." My wife said thank you and smiled with a little chuckle. Once we made it to the room, the nurse took my wife's blood pressure and told us that Dr. Melinda would be in to see us in a few minutes.

Soon after the nurse left, we heard a bunch of women right outside the door, talking. Jess and I could hear their entire conversation. It was Dr. Melinda, the nurse that showed us to the room, and about four other nurses outside the door talking. One of them said, "Dr. Melinda, I don't think Mrs. Randle started her chemo yet."

Dr. Melinda asked, "Why would you say that?"

The one nurse, along with the other four nurses, said, "She looks really good, not like a lot of patients we've had in the past, after they went through chemo."

Dr. Melinda asked, "What does she look like?"

One of the other nurses said, "She's tan, and she looks really in shape."

The other nurse said, "I remember her because her and her husband were really nice. She looks better now than when she first came here."

We heard Dr. Melinda respond with, "Okay then, let me go in here and see for myself."

When she walked in the room, her eyes went straight to my wife, and she had a look of disbelief. She asked Jess if she had started chemo treatment yet. My wife answered, "Yes, yes, I did. As a matter of fact, I am going on my seventh treatment." Dr. Melinda asked Jess what her routine was as far as eating and exercising. Jess explained everything to her, including the food she packed for lunch when she goes to her treatment, to all the different exercise she does. From walking, to kicking my butt in tennis, and walking in the morning and at night around our neighborhood. Dr. Melinda said, "Wow, you guys are very active."

We both said, "We try to be active as much as we can."

Dr. Melinda asked Jess if she could check her breast with the lump in it. She nodded yes. We didn't tell Dr. Melinda that the lump had shrunk. We wanted to see if she would notice a difference before we said anything, and she did right away. Before Dr. Melinda could ask, we told her about the two tumors on Jess's liver. She said, "Wow, that's really good news." She told us, right after Jess finished with her eighth treatment, that she would have to wait at least two months before she could have any surgery. We told her we completely understood because of the chemo. She told us to keep doing what we were doing and that Jess looked really good for being on her sixth treatment going to her seventh.

She was also very surprised that my wife had a head full of hair as well. We told her that Jess was on natural organic vitamins, and that was probably helping maintain her hair for so long. Dr. Melinda agreed, "Probably so, and that's a good thing you guys did all the research yourself." She told us to contact her office when we would like to set up an appointment two months after the eighth treatment. We left Dr. Melinda's office feeling good because we had gone through so much in a short amount of time; at least it felt like it was a short amount.

Three weeks flew by, and during that time, Jess had another CAT scan. The next day, Jess was going in for her seventh treatment. We met with Dr. Malata, and she told us she looked at my wife's scans, and the tumors on her liver had almost disappeared completely. There was still a lump in breast and an area in her lymph nodes under her arm. Dr. Thumalla said that the cancer was staying under her arm in one lymph node and not in any others. She said that was an unusual case that the cancer almost completely disappeared out of the liver and stayed just in the breast and lymph node and not spread anymore.

We took that as good news. Me being supportive for my wife, I was always nervous about Jess getting a CAT scan and going to Dr. Malata's office to hear the results. I was always like that and could not control that part, except with prayers. I always said a prayer every time Jess got a CAT scan and every time we went into the treatment area as well. That was what I did to stay calm. My grandmother taught me to always say a little prayer before you take any medicine or find yourself stuck in a difficult situation.

Well, we went into the treatment area, and it was full. One of the nurses told us we could go straight back to the middle of the room, back by the window. I don't know if they were looking at the chart to see when my wife was coming in or we were focusing on getting a window spot so much, but we always managed to get a chair right beside the window every time. I really don't know, but we both were very grateful for it. It wasn't as bad that day. A lot of people in our area were sleeping. The row to the right was a little chatty, but the left side row was pretty quiet.

When the nurse came over carrying the first cocktail bag for my wife, she asked Jess if the info on the bag of chemo was correct. My wife confirmed that it was correct. The nurse started to hook the bag up to the long metal pole when my wife asked her to put the sticky note on it for her. The nurse said, "Yes, of course I will." By now, the nurses were familiar with the sticky note. The nurse read it and gave my wife a big smile and put the sticky note on the bag.

After the nurse left, two other women asked Jess what was on the sticky note. My wife told them, "God's healing love." They were like "Okay!" and shook their heads up and down with a smile. A few minutes went by, and the same nurse came back with a basket of snacks and presented them to my wife. Jess explained, "No, thank you, I brought my own." The nurse went down the rest of the line asking people if they wanted any of the snacks. When she made it down the end to the last chair, there were no snacks left in the basket. I was so proud of my wife; she was sticking to the life style change of eating good foods.

Jess soon started pulling out her lunch, and a lot of eyes turned to see what she was pulling out of her little lunch bag. She pulled out some fruit, her celery, some organic peanut butter, some olives with cheese, and little beef cubes of sausages. A lot of the patients that could see my wife's lunch stopped eating their chips and cookies.

Later that night before bed, Jess was in the bathroom taking a shower, and I was sitting in the bed, reading. When I heard Jess get out of the shower about ten minutes later, she screamed. I jumped up and ran to the bathroom. Jess was standing there with a big clump of her hair in her left hand. She was almost in tears, staring at herself in the mirror. I told her, "Remember what the doctor said. Your hair would probably fall out going through chemo. It was just a matter of time."

She said with tears in her eyes, "I know, I just thought it wouldn't because I just had one more treatment to go."

I asked her what she wanted to do.

She decided firmly, "I don't want to walk around with patches of hair falling out of my head. Can you shave my hair off, please?"

I grabbed the clippers and started cutting a little at a time. I told her I always believed her head was shaped like a little potato. So now I finally got to see it. She started laughing because she didn't realize I had cut her a mohawk. We both couldn't stop laughing. I finished shaving the rest of her hair, joking the whole time, of course. My wife's head was not shaped like a potato; it was the shape of a little light bulb. We started laughing again. She giggled. "I really do have a light bulb–shaped head." She was staring in the mirror, laughing and rubbing her bald head. Jess was like, "Wow, I need to go get some more hats and scarves tomorrow." She was going to ask Abby to go with her the next day to go shopping before Bible study group that night. We went to bed rubbing on each other's bald heads, smiling at each other. (I have been shaving my head bald since after college.) My wife laid her head down on the pillow.

"So this is what the pillow feels like on your head?"

"Yep," I said, smiling back at her.

The next morning, my son and the doggies were in the kitchen when Jess walked out the bedroom. She had forgotten that she was bald, and my son questioned, "What happened to your hair?" Mia looked at Jess and turned her head to the side. Bear just sat there and looked at her like she was a stranger. Jess explained to Anthony Jr., "It was falling out last night, so I had your dad shave the rest of it off." After Mia and Bear heard Jess's voice, they walked up to her wagging their tails.

After breakfast, Jess called Abby and explained about her hair falling out last night. She asked her if she would go with her to find some nice hats and scarves. Abby was happy to go and asked Jess if she wanted to go by the wig store. Jess decided, "No, no wigs for me, just hats." That night at Bible study, everyone was looking at Jess as though they just came to the realization that Jess really did have breast cancer. The only ones who looked at her normally were Donna V., Abby, and Alex.

Donna V. suggested to Jess she come in for an energy session tomorrow and asked if she thought I would like to do an energy session as well. Jess said, "I think it would do him some good to get his energy lined back up." When Jess finally asked me to do it, I told her no because it was for her, not for me. She told me we both were in this together, and she thought it would be good for me to get my energy lined back up. I gave in and told her and Donna V. that I would do it.

That night during the middle of Bible study, I could tell it was still bothering Abby about Jess going through what she was going through. I talked to Abby and the other Bible study group members about how strong Jess was and that we were going to get through everything just fine because we had our whole Bible study group praying for us. Abby's eyes started to water up, and she said she had to go and check on her son, who was sleeping in the back room.

After Bible study, I told Abby that Jess would be fine. She was doing great on eating the right foods and staying away from sugars and processed foods. I also told her that the spots on her liver were almost gone and that she still was doing treatment for the spot in her breast and lymph node. She felt better after I had talked to her more about Jess. Jess had told her too that she was doing good and feeling good.

That night walking home from Abby's house, we walked around the neighborhood twice, talking about traveling to a beach somewhere and vacationing at a beach house. All the stars were out that night, and my wife was pointing out the Big Dipper and the Little Dipper to me. I told her I said a prayer for her to be able to be on a beach or go to an island so she could relax and it would help with her healing. I told her she was a water baby, and I was a land baby. She started laughing, and then I put her in a headlock while we were walking. It didn't take much to put her in a headlock because my wife's head was so tiny now that she was bald like me.

I let her go out of the headlock because a neighbor was driving by, and I didn't want them to think I was beating up a neighborhood kid. My wife started laughing again because she was thinking the same thing. We were down the street from the house, and it was around ten o'clock. I told Jess "Let's say another prayer" as we walked to the courtyard area of the house. This time we held hands and faced each other. We said our prayers while looking up at the stars, and then we walked into the house.

The next day, we went over to see Donna V. for Jess's energy session, and I had totally forgot about me going through an energy session with Donna V. After Jess went through her session, I was ready to go home. Donna V. refused to let me go. "No, you have an appointment today as well." I told her I had completely forgot. I suggested to her and Jess that we make it for some other time. They both said *no* at the same time. There I was, this six-foot, four-inch guy being pressured by two five-foot, two-inch women. That wasn't cool at all. They were looking at me like "You big baby." My wife was pushing me through the door with Donna V. pulling me by my right arm. I told both of them, "Okay, okay, I'll do this."

I went ahead and walked in Donna's little room. It was nice and peaceful in there, a sort of a calming effect. She asked me a couple of questions, and then she had me take off my shoes and socks. I told her, "I am going to take off my shoes, but I don't know about my socks."

She questioned me, "Why not your socks?"

I responded with, "Because of all the pressure you and my wife just put me through to come in here, my feet started sweating." Donna V. laughed and assured me it would be ok. I told her, "Okay,

I am not being held liable if you pass out in here and hit the ground choking." Really, I was trying to stall so she would kick me out or stop the session. No such luck. She didn't kick me out. She told me to relax while she stood at my feet. I didn't tell Jess or Donna V. my head was hurting that day from my sinuses. It was really throbbing, especially when I lay down.

Donna V. told me to take three deep breaths and relax. When I closed my eyes, the last thing I remember was Donna V. down by the bottom of my feet. About three minutes later, I could feel the heat from Donna V.'s body standing to my right side. Then she was by the left side of my head, where my head was hurting from the sinus migraine. The side of my body and my face started sweating. All I could think was, *Wow, Donna V. is giving off a lot of body heat.* I could feel her hand on the side of my face, like the way my grandmother used to touch me when I had a headache as a kid. Donna V. was following the same pattern or routine my grandmother did to rub my head and then between and around my eyes. Then the hand paused over my head and stayed there. My grandmother stopped her hand in the same spot because she would say more prayers before she moved her hand from over my head. My headache stopped. Donna V. had stopped my headache by doing the same thing my grandmother used to do.

I felt Donna V. move over to my right side because I felt even more heat. It felt like, for some reason, she was standing on something because this person was tall, and the person to my left was short and still standing there. I was thinking that Donna had let someone in the room or something. This person, or Donna V., laid their hands on my shoulder, and I started sweating all over again. Then the hand removed itself. I couldn't wait to get out of this meditative state or relaxation state I was in because I was going to tell her about all the heat she was creating around me.

Donna V. told me to take three deep breaths and move my fingers, then my hands, and then my toes. I started moving my hands, my feet, and my toes like she said and slowly opened my eyes. She asked me how I was feeling. I told her I was feeling great, besides all the sweating on my right and my left sides from the heat she was producing from moving around my head. She told me it wasn't her. I was confused and said, "What?"

She explained, "I was standing down here by your feet the whole time." She asked in a scared and excited voice, "Who was it, and what did you see?" She told me, "There were two hazy-like figures, one to your left and one to your right." She confessed that she could see the figures in the room but couldn't make out who it was. She could just see waves. I was like, "Waves?"

Donna V. explained, "Yes, like heat waves, you know, like on a hot day. You're driving down the highway, and you look further down the street, and it's all wavy from the heat." She said there was two of them by my head. The one came first by my left side, then about five or ten minutes later, the other one showed up.

Normally I would have jumped up and run out of the room at that point. But you would have to know Donna V. She's the real deal when it comes to being very spiritual. She helped Jess so much throughout the year we were very grateful for her and her friendship. I told her thank you for the session, and I was feeling so much better. I asked her, "So this is what my wife feels like after every session?"

She answered, "Jess tells me that after every session, she feels really relaxed."

Donna V. and I walked back into the waiting area, and Jess asked me how I felt.

I told her, "Great."

She said excitedly, "See, I told you it would help you. Do you feel like everything is flowing in your body correctly?"

I told her, "Yes, it does."

We paid Donna V. and both gave her a big hug goodbye. I had to bend down because she was so short and so tiny. I told Jess I would tell her some more about my session once we got in the car. On the way out the door, everything was super bright outside. It was around five o'clock in the evening, and it was so bright it looked like the sun had just come up. I couldn't wait to get to the car because I had tinted windows. Jess had to hold my hand and guide me to the car and then to the driver side door.

Once I got in, I had to wait for my eyes to adjust before I could start driving. Jess didn't like driving my car because it was lowered, and she couldn't avoid the potholes fast enough. Once I started driving, I began explaining everything to Jess about what had happened during my session. She told me out of about eight sessions she had so far, that only happened to her once. She said, "That was good that they showed up right away to help you."

I questioned, "They?"

She asked, "Donna V. didn't explain it to you?"

"Explain what?"

She explained, "These are people or spirits in our life that watch over us. It could be a relative that you were close to or a pet even."

"A pet?" I asked.

"Yes, a pet."

Jess told me the story of a lady having a pet when she was little, and it passed away. It came to visit her during her session. I argued sweetly, "Well, Donna V. told me she can't make out anything and that it looks like heat waves." Jess told me she could make this one out because it was jumping around like it was happy and playing.

"Trust me," she said, "Donna V. has show dogs, and she has been around them her whole life." Jess explained to me, "The reason Donna V. didn't tell you a lot is because she didn't want you to freak out and jump up off the table."

I was thinking to myself, I would have done more than that. I would have jumped off the table and threw my wife the keys on my way out the door and ran all the way home nonstop. My wife wouldn't have caught me until I made it to the highway. But for my wife, I stayed pretty calm for the most part. Plus, I was calm when the waves or spirits were there, so it all worked out.

I told my wife I was very thankful for the energy alignment and that I felt like I had a lot more energy and my headache was gone. I knew the next question from my wife was coming. I think she was building up to it. She asked me, "Who do you think the two people were at each side of your head?"

I told her I knew it was my grandmother right after Donna V. told me it wasn't her. "But the person standing on the other side, I don't know who that person was."

My wife said proudly, "I knew it was your grandmother because you told me plenty of times how she cured your migraines for you without any medicine. Who do you think the other person was?" I told her it could have been my uncle or my grandfather. "I am glad you got to have a session with Donna V. because you got to see what I feel like right after."

The next day we received a phone call from our boss, Lenny. He said he wanted to talk to us about something that was very important. He asked first, "How are you two doing?" We told him we were doing great, and the two tumors on Jess's liver were almost gone. We also explained everything to him about her breast and lymph nodes. We told him that Jess had one more treatment to go, treatment number 8. Lenny said that was great news and that he knew she was going to pull through everything okay.

He said the reason he was calling was that we had been gone a little over a year. We both said at the same time, "A year? It hasn't been that long."

He said, "Yeah, it's been a little over a year."

We were like, "*Wow!*" We both didn't realize how time had flown by so fast.

He began explaining, "Well, I wanted to offer Jess a job. So, Jess, how about it?"

She responded, puzzled, "How about what?"

He laughed a little, "How about you being my deputy so I can train you to be my backup for my position?"

Jess was frozen on the phone. She didn't know what to say except, "You're kidding, right?" with a serious tone. "Lenny, is this a joke? Because I don't think it's very funny at all."

Lenny quickly answered, "No, no, it's not a joke. I am being serious."

She looked at me, "What do I do?"

I told her to take it.

Lenny interrupted us and said there was a couple of stipulations.

"Okay, what are the stipulations, Lenny?"

He responded, "You guys would have to probably sell your house in Vegas and move to El Paso."

I said, "Okay, done."

My wife looked at me. "Are you sure?"

I replied, "You're always sacrificing for me and my jobs, so this is the least I can do for you."

Then Lenny said there was one more thing.

"Really, Lenny, one more thing?"

He started laughing again. "You will have to leave the program because it would be a conflict of interest if you both are on the program with Jess being in charge."

I understood this minor technicality and asked if he had another program I could go to. Lenny informed us, "We think you would be a good fit to be on the radar testing team."

I asked him about all the details, and he told me that it would take place in Hawaii. First, I had to travel to some other location for some additional training. I asked excitedly, "Okay then, when do I start?" He asked when Jess's last treatment was scheduled. I told him, "In two weeks." He told us both he would need me in two to three months after Jess's last chemo. Jess could take her time and start in El Paso when she was ready to come back. We both agreed these were good options, but I had a question for him. "How long will I be over in Hawaii?" He told me he didn't know how long or when I would go over because he didn't have the schedule of the timeline for everything to take place. He said the company was still working out the logistics of everything.

After getting the good news from Lenny and we hung up with him, I told Jess that I had said a prayer about going over to Hawaii or some island beach when we were at treatment. I told her I thought it would help in her healing process to go relax and enjoy the beach. I kept a mental picture of us walking on the beach together just relaxing and enjoying ourselves. She was blown away when I told her. She grabbed my hand. "Come here, I need to show you something …" She turned on the TV. "Watch this." She showed me all the TV programs she had recorded, including shows from HGTV, *Hawaii Life*, and one about buying houses by the beach.

We both had to sit down for a minute and thank God for this blessing. She was almost in tears about the timing of everything. She told me she had asked the universe a question last week, and she didn't think the answer would come so quickly. She asked about our jobs and where they would put us in the company to work because she had no desire to travel back overseas again.

"It seems like we got our answers all at once," I told her.

"We pretty much did," she agreed.

I took her hat off her little head and rubbed small circles on the top and told her, "This is how our wishes really came true." She started laughing. I giggled. "Liiiight bulb."

We were getting closer to Jess's eighth and final cocktail treatment. Her hair had started growing back fast. We noticed it was growing back reddish brown with gray on each side, like the comic book hero Dr. Steve Richards of the Fantastic Four. It was really cool because my wife was a brunet. Plus, there were now these big curls in her hair, when before her hair was straight and long. Jess still wore her hats though because she said she paid a lot of money for those hats, and they were not going to go to waste. She did look cool and really cute in her hats too.

We were into the week of Jess's eighth treatment, and we felt like we were at the finish line. We went in the treatment center to Dr. Malata's office. The nurse had weighed Jess. She had lost about twenty pounds total. The nurse was a little concerned, but my wife told her she had completely stopped eating sugar. The nurse told her that would explain the weight loss, but she advised Jess not to lose any more. My wife told her she wasn't planning on losing any more, and she liked the weight she was at.

The nurse soon left. Dr. Malata walked in with a big smile on her face and asked us how we were doing. We told her we were doing well and happy that this was the last treatment. Dr. Malata had to explain to us that this would be the last of the cocktails of all the chemo drugs, but it wouldn't be the last treatment. My wife and I stared at Dr. Malata, trying to get a grasp on what she was talking about. She was nervous because I think she realized she never said anything to us about more treatments after the eighth one. My wife had this look of disbelief, and she questioned, "What do you mean it's not my last treatment?" Dr. Malata quickly explained that Jess would not have to take all the drugs like she was doing but that she would have to take two of them for a year or two. Then down to one drug for a year or two. She said it was normal for patients to be on a very low dose for five years or so just as a preventative measure. Once there was no sign of the cancer at the five-year mark, the treatments could stop, and she would just come in for regular checkups.

Now this caught us a little off guard. We decided at the beginning that it would be in our best interest, no matter what was said throughout the rest of the doctor visits, not to get upset and put ourselves in a negative state of mind. We started this whole process, my wife and I, by not watching the news on TV or reading the paper. If we wanted to watch a movie, it would have to be a comedy or a love story.

Dr. Malata finished explaining that my wife could take a small break after her last cocktail for about three to four weeks, but she would still have to come in for checkups on her time off from treatment. We both thanked Dr. Malata for all her patience and understanding. We also thanked her for always entering the room with a smile on her face. She told us it was us, this whole time, that put a smile on her face because we stuck together and Jess never gave up. Dr. Malata informed us, "It's very rare to see couples, let alone a partner, be so dedicated during times like this." We talked a little more with Dr. Malata before we headed over to the treatment room across the hallway.

When we walked in, the nurse said they were full on the left side, and the middle of the room was full as well. She said we had to go to the right side in the back by the window. We walked over to the right side, trailing the nurse, when we both heard a familiar voice. It was the lady that was on the ground screaming that time, but this day she was laughing and talking to everyone. She spoke to us as we passed by her chair and even complimented Jess on what a nice hat she was wearing. Jess said thank you and sat her bag down next to her chair in the corner by the window. We both noticed that the screaming lady had brought a friend with her to support her this time. We knew that was what she needed before but didn't have, someone there to support her.

Everyone else in the area was pleasant, and it wasn't as noisy over in the area as it had been in the past. Jess's nurse came back with her bags of cocktail and hooked them up to the pole. Jess handed her the sticky note to put on her bag. The screaming lady noticed the note and asked my wife what the note said. Before my wife could answer, the nurse said "God's healing love" and smiled at Jess. Screaming lady said, "Oh, okay," and then smiled. I grabbed Jess's computer for her, and we started looking up the different islands in Hawaii. We were both excited and amazed and thankful all at the same time.

After we left the treatment center, I asked Jess what she wanted to do today. She said happily, "Let's go play tennis." I started having flashbacks of the last time we played tennis, but I decided I was going to beat her today, cocktail or no cocktail. I told her after we left the house, "I am in competition mode now, so get ready." She started laughing. I told her I was completely serious.

Once we arrived at the tennis court, I grabbed the rackets out of the back seat along with the tennis balls. I started walking up the sidewalk. Jess ran up beside me and pushed me off the sidewalk to break my concentration. I told her it wasn't going to work. We got on the court and started stretching. I asked her if she was ready. She said, "Let's do this." My wife kicked my butt so bad I told her I needed to go see a chiropractor after the beating I just took. She started laughing. I was hurting so bad I couldn't even laugh. I felt like I was just hit by a runaway truck.

That following week, my son left for basic training. His departure had been delayed. It was hard seeing him leave because I didn't have anyone to watch football with or talk about sport cars. Jess would watch football with me but would always fall asleep. I could always thank football for putting Jess to sleep when she wouldn't sit still and needed the rest. Jess was doing good. She had her routine down like clockwork. She would get up in the morning and would feed Mia and Bear. Then she and I would go for a four- to six-mile bike ride. If she was sore from the bike ride, we would go for a walk around the neighborhood or go to the nearby park and walk. After our exercise, we would return home and start breakfast.

I wanted her to get in a routine because I just had this feeling that I would have to leave sooner than Lenny had stated on the phone. Our company was like that; some things would move fast, and some things would move slow, depending on the priority at the time. It made me feel a little better knowing she would still be exercising and taking care of herself while I was away.

It was time for Jess to start going back to treatment. We preferred to call it maintenance instead of treatment. I went in with her. The time and day she was scheduled, there wasn't a lot of patients in the treatment area. She would still have to do blood work because of the spot in her right breast, which was still shrinking, by the way, and the lymph node under her arm. Jess told me I didn't have to go with her to maintenance. I asked her if she was sure. She assured me she would be okay because it was only going to be about an hour and thirty minutes. Plus, she was going to meet up with Abby and go shopping afterward. I was fine with it then because I realized she wasn't getting a lot of friend time with her female friends. I was very happy to hear that she and Abby were going to go shopping.

About an hour or two after Jess left, my cell phone rang, and it was Lenny. He had called to tell me they would need me to come back to work soon, and I would be traveling to Boston, Massachusetts, to start on a project. I told him Jess had started the maintenance part of her treatment and that she would still need surgery later. He asked me when I would be able to leave for Boston. I told him I could go in about three weeks just to make sure everything was okay with Jess before I left her by herself. He understood and told me he would send me some forms to fill out to reactivate my clearance. He would have his administrative assistant, Mary, to schedule my plane ticket and hotel reservation for me.

After I hung up with Lenny, I checked the calendar just to make sure I had enough time to see my son when he returned from basic training, and I did. I would still have two weeks at home when he returned. Now I just had to let Jess know about me leaving in three weeks. I didn't know why, but I was so nervous about telling her, and she already knew I would have to go back to work. I think it was just me. I was nervous about leaving her. I knew some couples only could be around each other but so long and then they'd need a break from each other. My wife and I loved and enjoyed being around each other. We were each other's best friend. So you can see why it was going to be hard to tell her and for me to leave.

I talked to Jess when she came home, and she was good with me leaving. She said, "At least you're not going overseas."

I agreed. "You know what, you're right, I never looked at it that way."

She added, "Plus, I could come and visit you anytime."

It was funny because I thought she would be the nervous one, but it was me that was worried and didn't want to leave. Like I said before, my wife is a strong woman. But the days she was not so strong, I was there for her.

A week had gone by so quickly, and my son was back home from army basic training. He was glad to see us, and we were glad to see him. I gave him a big hug, told him I packed his suitcase with all the clothes he left behind, and told him to get out. My wife started laughing. My son looked at me, like, "Really, Pops? How are you going to give me a hug and then kick me out?"

I explained to him, "That wasn't a hug for 'Welcome home,' that was a hug for 'Goodbye, you're moving out.'"

After that we were all laughing. Mia and Bear were running around playing because all of us were laughing so much.

The week came for me to leave. I had my ticket in hand and was ready to fly out. My son had to work that morning, so he couldn't come to the airport. We said our goodbyes before he went to work. Mia and Bear knew I was leaving because they had seen the suitcases the night before. Mia wouldn't eat anything that morning. Bear was sad, but he wasn't going to let that get in the way of food time. He ran straight to his dish and buried his face in his bowl. I tried to comfort Mia before I left, but I was running short on time getting to the airport. Jess told me that Mia would be okay. We needed to get going to beat all the traffic to the airport.

Once we arrived at the airport, Jess walked in with me to the ticket counter and then over to the security check area for all the gates. I told her it was very hard for me to leave her, and I knew she felt the same way. I knew she was being strong for the both of us. I told her that I loved her, and I would call her once I landed in Boston. She held my hand, and I could tell she didn't want to let it go. Once I made it through the metal detector, I couldn't see her because she was so short, but I waved anyway. I figured she could see my big hand waving. Jess was still standing there because she saw my hand. She jumped a little, just enough for me to see the top of her head and her hand waving.

As soon as I got on the plane, I called her because I wanted to make sure she got out of the airport okay. She told me that she had no problem leaving the airport, and it was a good thing we left when we did because there was a traffic jam going into the airport. I was quiet that whole flight. There was an older gentleman that sat beside me trying to make conversation, but I wasn't in the mood to talk. As soon as he got up to go to the bathroom, I put my shades and my headphones on and went to sleep.

Once I made it to Boston, which was freezing cold, I grabbed my rental car and was off to the hotel in Burlington, Massachusetts. I had finally arrived at the hotel. I couldn't wait to get to my room and out of the cold. I wanted to call Jess while I was driving, but the rental car didn't have Bluetooth, and I was using the GPS on my phone. I got to my room and put all my clothes away and called Jess. We both instantly got excited just hearing each other's voice.

I went right into husband slash best friend slash caregiver mode. I asked her if she exercised today and what type of exercise she did. I asked her what she ate for breakfast and lunch. I wanted to make sure she was taking her medicine she needed to take before bed. She told me to calm down and take a deep breath. I told her I was calm, but I really wasn't. So I did like she said and took some deep breaths and calmed myself down. Jess asked, "Okay, are you good now?"

I assured her, "Yeah, I'm good now."

Jess told me not to worry about her so much because worrying didn't fix or help anything. She encouraged, "Focus on the job and time will go by fast. The next time we see each other, we will be in Hawaii." She told me if she needed anything, Anthony Jr. was right there with her. I was a little more relieved then.

The month up in Boston went by fast, and the next thing you know, I was flying down to El Paso, Texas. I met with Lenny as soon as I arrived, and he gave me more information on how the movement would go as far as going over to Kauai. I was in El Paso for about two weeks, and then the team and I flew over to Kauai with the equipment we were working on. Once we arrived, we looked around for housing. I was able to find a nice little condo close to the beach. It was right around all the resorts, restaurants, and shopping areas for Jess. I figured she could easily walk or ride a bike around. She could go to all the different resorts blending in with the vacationers and enjoy swimming at the different resort pools. It was about three weeks until we could get a schedule that the team could agree on. Once I had a set schedule, I quickly made arrangements to fly Jess over.

The day came when I finally picked her up at the airport in Kauai. I was so excited I probably only slept about three or four hours the night before I had to pick her up. I left the condo like three hours early. One, because I was excited, and two, because I didn't want to get lost or be late to pick up my beautiful little wife. Once I got to the airport, it was like no airport I had ever seen. See, when the team and I flew in, we landed at the far end of the airport with the military around 2:00 a.m. We really couldn't see the airport at all, just the runway.

The airport was small but very nice and really open with one baggage terminal. There were two vendors at the baggage claim area where you could buy flower leis that went around your neck. The other vendor was selling the leis that went around your head. I bought my wife the one that was made out of these beautiful purple flowers. They had a nice smell to them that wasn't too overwhelming. I wanted it to take my wife's breath away as soon as I placed them on her neck. I was tired from working the day before. I was more excited to see my wife, so the tiredness really didn't bother me as much.

Once her plane landed, I couldn't wait to hug her and give her a kiss. It felt like forever since we had seen each other though it had only been about two months. When I saw her, we both made eye contact as soon as she came around the corner of the small hallway. She ran over to me. I walked faster over to her, trying not to run anyone over as I was trying to get to my wife. I picked her up and hugged her. I almost forgot I had the lei in my hand. She asked me what that nice smell was. I showed it to her, and she loved it. I put it around her neck and went to get her bags.

As we left the airport, I couldn't help but notice the dark circles around her eyes and asked her if she was okay. Jess told me she was so excited to come over to the island that she didn't get any sleep. I grabbed her hands with my right hand and held both her hands all the way to the resort area where I was staying. I let her know, as we were getting out of the car, that I went to the grocery store two days ago after work. I tried to find as much organic food as possible. She told me she was sure I got plenty for us for a couple of days.

We finally made it into the condo, and she loved it, especially the large balcony overlooking two resorts and the blue water of the ocean. We stood out on the balcony while she just absorbed the rays of the sunshine and the cool breeze of the ocean. Jess asked me, "Is the breeze like this all the time?"

I told her it was most of the time. "When the breeze is not blowing, it gets really hot here on the island." I added, "I just turn on the ceiling fans and put the floor fan directly on me. If you don't have the fan on you directly, you will wake up in a pile of sweat."

There was no AC in any of the condos where I stayed because the ocean breeze was pretty much constant through the day and at night. Jess was so tired I told her to lay down for a while. After her nap, I would take her around and show her the different beaches and shopping areas. I told her I would lay down with her so she would sleep better. I closed all the front blinds because people would actually walk by and look in your condo, especially little kids running back and forth on the front deck. I left all the blinds open in the back by the patio. I placed the fan in between the bedroom and the living room so it would pull the ocean breeze through the condo. We slept for about three or four hours.

When we woke up, I ordered some food from the local well-known restaurant Keoki's Paradise, on the south side of the island and happened to be right across the street. I knew she would like the hamburger I had ordered her because it was a Hawaiian-style hamburger and was very popular. It was called a Rancher's Burger. It was made with local grass fed beef, house smoked bacon with Swiss cheese, arugula, tomato jam, and roasted garlic aioli on a sweet Hawaiian bun. Just describing this hamburger makes me want one right now.

Jess smelled the hamburger as soon as I walked in the door with it, and she attacked this burger like there was no tomorrow. She said only four words after the very first bite, "Wow, this is good!" Now normally this was how our eating routine would go whenever we ate any type of meal, especially hamburgers. Now, I am a big guy, six feet, four inches and around 285 pounds, built like a large linebacker. My wife is five feet, two inches, 125 pounds, and built like a little gymnast. Every time she ate, she always, I mean always, had leftovers. So of course I thought this time was no different. Jess was almost halfway finished with her burger. I just knew she was going to slow down very soon because she had finished her fries already.

I wasn't even halfway finished with my burger because I was so busy looking at her eat her burger. She was eating that burger like it was the last burger on the island and she had it all to herself. I was literally sitting there, watching my wife eat this burger in turbo-speed mode. There was no sign of her slowing down. I looked over at her again. It was like she got her second wind and started eating the other half of her burger. Up in my head I was saying, *Okay, short fry, you're messing up our routine here.* (That was the nickname I had for her in college.) I looked over at Jess after she ate the rest of her burger, and I was still working on my burger.

She said, completely satisfied, "That was one of the best and healthiest burgers I ever ate." I told her she ate her burger like a wild mountain lion would eat a poor little helpless deer. I told her I felt bad for that burger; it had no chance. She started laughing and stole some of my fries. I had to get up and move to the living room from the dining table while bear hugging my plastic container. She was still laughing the whole time and still trying to get to my fries. Finally, she stopped reaching for my fries and said, "I need to go to the oval office." I told her she was nasty, and I was still trying to finish my food. She started laughing again while walking to the bathroom.

A few minutes later, my burger started to smell a little nasty, and I remembered that my wife was in the bathroom. I screamed at her, "Hey, spray something … anything … you're stinky!"

She laughed some more and said, "You don't really smell me out there."

I screamed back, "OH YES, I CAN!"

She was like, "REALLY?"

I told her, "This condo is only so big, plus the breeze from the front door is bringing your smell into the living room. It's making my gourmet burger taste sour."

She laughed even louder, and what followed her laughter was a trail of untimed farts. She said, "I'm sorry. I can't help it. You're making me laugh!" And then she would let out another one.

Finally, I started laughing because they started sounding like a broken whistle. She finally found some air freshener and sprayed after she walked out of the bathroom. We were both still laughing about it as she asked me about the rest of the food places around the area. I told her that she needed to try the fish tacos tomorrow. I would drive her along the south side of the island, and we could stop along the way to walk on the beach.

The next day we got up and made breakfast. Then we went for a short walk around the condo area and down to the beach. It was only a handful of people out that morning, so we sat on the edge of the beach in the grass. We talked about what type of house we wanted to buy once we moved to El Paso. I decided that we would pay for movers to help her since I wasn't able to be there. I told her hopefully Anthony Jr. would be there to help as well. She assured me she would get everything taken care of as far as moving.

We got up after about an hour and started walking again through some more resort areas. Then we got in the car and drove along the south side of the island to get some fish tacos. After we got our delicious fish tacos, I drove down to another beach that the local islanders always went to. We arrived, and I could tell that Jess really loved this beach. I told her I passed this beach every morning going to work. She asked, "It must look really nice early in the morning." I told her it looked peaceful in the early morning.

As we walked down the beach, I had this weird feeling that someone was following us. I asked Jess, "Do you get the feeling someone is following us?"

She looked around. "I don't see anyone."

I said to her, "I don't see them, but I can feel them."

She suggested, "Let's walk a little and then stop to see if you feel the same way." I agreed. We walked a little farther and then we stopped. "Do you still feel the same way?"

"Yes, I do."

We both looked down the beach, up ahead of us on the beach, but still didn't see anything. So I looked out into the ocean, and I noticed a big, large dark spot in the water. I grabbed Jess. "Look! What is that?"

"I don't know."

I pulled her. "Let's start walking." We did, and the large dark circle started moving with us. We stopped again, and it stopped with us. We started walking, and it started moving with us. I mean, it was moving right beside us and keeping pace with our every step. It followed us for about a hundred yards, and then we figured it out. It was a large sea turtle the whole time.

We were so excited. It was our first time seeing a sea turtle up close. I had lost track of the time and realized I had to get Jess out of the sun before she started burning. We made our way back to the car and drove to the condo. The whole way there, we talked about the turtle and how amazing that was that it was following us down the beach like that. My wife looked over at me and asked, "Do you think that turtle could feel our positive energy and that's why it was following us?" I told her either that or the turtle was thinking, "Wow, I wish they would stop hogging the beach and following me so I can lay my eggs somewhere." Jess started laughing and said that could be true as well. She thanked me for taking her out that day. Dr. Malata told her to get plenty of sun while she was over here because the sun provided instant vitamin D for her body. I was so happy she was happy being there, and something told me that this would play a big part in her healing.

You know how sometimes you aren't thinking of anything and it feels like someone comes up and whispers an idea in your ear? It's a totally different voice and not your own. Well, that was happening a lot since that night of that dream and walking out of the closet the next morning. So now, I always make it a point to listen to this voice because it hasn't steered me wrong yet.

That night we decided to sit out on the patio for a while before we went to bed and talked about our house situation in El Paso. I told her I thought we should just look for a house to rent and not buy anything right away. I didn't want Jess to put a lot of stress on her body trying to move along with trying to buy a house. I told her it would be much easier and quicker to rent at first. She agreed and said she didn't want to mentally wear herself out, especially going into a new job. I felt like this would be a good time to pick my wife's brain on what type of house she wanted, as far as appliances, how many bedrooms and bathrooms.

Jess started off by saying she wanted a modern-style home around 2,400 to 3,100 square feet. She said she would like at least four bedrooms, and we could turn one into an office, and a large gourmet kitchen with an exhaust fan that actually filtered the smoke to the outside. She wanted a large master bathroom with a fireplace. Not just any fireplace, one of those you could change the color of the flames with glass at the bottom. She also wanted a large living room with an even bigger fireplace than the one in the master bedroom. She wanted a good-sized backyard.

I told her, "You really put a lot of thought into this house." She told me she had a vision of what she wanted the house to look like all the way to the interior and exterior wall color. I couldn't wait to see this house come to life. She told me about the furniture she had been looking at in different magazines. She cut out some of the pictures and hung them up. I was like, "Wow! This house up in your head is going to be really nice, and I can't wait to find it!"

That next morning, me and Jess walked over to the Marriot resort and had breakfast. We never had breakfast by the beach before. It was really peaceful because you could hear the waves crashing up against the rocks and the ocean breeze hitting the surrounding palm trees. I had to work the next two days while she was there. She told me she had a feeling I wouldn't be able to take off the whole time she was there, but she understood because my job was why I was there to begin with. So the rest of the day we just relaxed and enjoyed each other's company.

The first day I went to work, Jess told me she fell asleep on the balcony reading a book, and drool was running down the side of her mouth onto the balcony floor. She told me when she woke up it was a small swimming pool of drool on the side of her chair. She thought she must have been asleep for a couple of hours, because she felt dehydrated. I informed her, "The reason you felt dehydrated was because of all the slobber you left on the balcony. That's where all your fluids went." We both started laughing. I asked her if she drank a lot of water. She assured me she did because she had gone for a long walk right after I left for work that morning.

The next day Jess went shopping and walked around the different art galleries. She managed to collect a couple of necklaces that were made out of the local seashells from one of the resorts. Sometimes my wife could get caught up in the moment of shopping, so I questioned her about what she had to eat all day. Before she could answer, I joked, "You know how you get with your shopping … You will be looking around and see something 'Oooo, somethin' shiny' and forget all about eating."

She started laughing. "No, I remembered to eat. I couldn't help but to eat after smelling all the different foods that were being cooked during lunch."

She had gotten another hamburger with some calamari and a salad for dinner. I asked her if she brought me something. She said seriously, "No, I didn't get you anything to eat this time."

I looked at her, like, "Really?"

"I am just kidding … I got you a burger and a salad."

I told her that was exactly what I was thinking about getting when I got off from work, and she got me one anyway. It was awesome.

That night we talked, and she could tell right away I was feeling a little down because I had to take her to the airport before I went to work the next morning. I told her I felt sad, like instantly, when I knew she had to leave. She told me she felt the same way; she just hid it really well. It was a little comforting when she told me that everything was going to be okay, and she would be coming back over in a couple of weeks. I still felt a little sad though. It had never gotten easier for me to be away from her as a husband, a best friend, and a caregiver. I always wanted to be there to protect her from anything and everything. But like my grandmother always said, "Sometimes you have to put it in God's hands."

The next morning, I drove her to the Lihue Airport. We sat in the car for a while in short-term parking. I think we both were trying to comfort each other and to make sure we were both going to be okay until her next trip. I told Jess I would be okay because I had to go straight to work, and the long drive down the coast of the island would help ease my mind. She said she had a lot to do once she got home, and that would keep her busy as well. I think we needed that from each other before we got out of the car.

It was like getting a pep talk from a coach. I could see Jess as a coach saying, "Everything is gonna be okay. Now rub some dirt on it and get back out there!" My wife always described me as the Motivator in our family unit. She keeps encouraging me to get into motivational speaking. I keep telling her I just look at it as being a good supporter for my family.

As we walked to the ticket counter, reality set in for me that she was leaving. I started to have that pain in my chest and that lump in my throat. I couldn't really tell how my wife was doing because she was in travel mode at that point, changing her seats around, weighing her luggage, and getting her tickets. Afterward, we went and sat down on one of the concrete benches that was located by the terminal entrance. Jess asked me how I was holding up. I told her I was holding up pretty well. Which I was. I was just a little sad because I was going to miss her. We sat there and watched the people go through the terminal. We held hands until it was time for her to go through her terminal.

I stood and watched until she went through the metal detector. I couldn't see her anymore until she jumped up in the air, waving her hand. All I could do was wave and hope she could see me. I then walked across the street because I had about a little over an hour drive to work. Really, the speed limit made the drive that long. The speed limit on the whole island was between fifteen and thirty-five miles per hour. The only thing that stopped you from falling asleep at the wheel was the nice scenery and trying to avoid hitting wild chickens trying to cross the road. It was always a scenic drive though, no matter where you went on the island.

On my way back to work, I received a phone call from one of the guys on my team telling me I didn't have to come in, and they had covered my shift. I told them they couldn't have called at a better time because I was getting close to the resort area where we stayed. I stopped by one of the local grocery stores on the way to the condo to stock up on some more food for the workweek. Afterward, I drove back to the condo so I could start prepping my meals for the week.

Right after I was done cooking, I sat down, and instantly my thoughts started running. It was almost like my brain was running wild with no remote to control it. I put my hands over my head to stop all the negative thoughts from fully taking control of me. The worst part wasn't everything negative that was running through my head; it was when the thoughts included my wife. The first thought that popped up in my head was, *Is she going to be okay on the plane? What if something happens to the plane, and I wasn't there to protect her?* I promised her mom I would take care of her daughter. I even started questioning her health. Was she getting better? She looked like she lost a lot of weight. She wasn't eating enough. She wasn't exercising enough like she was supposed to. You should have made her rest more. Finally, I had to scream in my head, "Stop! Just stop!"

All of a sudden, the negative thoughts stopped attacking me. I didn't know how long I could keep them at bay until it happened again. So I grabbed a piece of paper and a pen, and I drew a line down the middle. On the left side I put True at the top of the page. On the right side, I put False. Beside the word False, I wrote Brain to signify my brain was creating things that were nonexistent. I started with my first question, "Is your wife safe?" I put a slash under True. Then I asked the second question, "Is your wife healthy in your eyes?" I put a slash under True. Then the third question, "Is your wife taking good care of herself?" I put another slash under True. My fourth question was, "Are you doing the very best you can to help your wife with her healing process?" I put another slash under True.

I sat back in the chair, looked at the paper, and realized my brain was creating things that were not there. I was creating fear, fear of things that had not happened and might never happen. At that moment, I realized I was letting my brain control me and not me controlling my brain. It was around 9:00 p.m. when Jess texted me she had landed in Seattle, and she had to go right to her next flight. I texted back, "Okay, I love you very much." She said the same and asked me how I was doing. I told her I was doing good. She also told me I needed to go to bed since I had to work the next day. She knew I really didn't sleep when she, or our son, traveled. I told her I would try to get some sleep.

I went back to trying to figure out how to calm my brain down and stop those attacks I was having. I started thinking about everything I was grateful for in my life. When I said how grateful I was for my wife, I instantly started having flashbacks of her having the courage to go to A&P school when she never even worked on a plane before. She finished second in her class out of twenty-five guys who had prior mechanic backgrounds in the air force. She bravely moved to California to work on UAVs and was one of the top female mechanics at her company. When we almost lost everything, the house, the cars, I mean everything, she opened an eBay account and started selling all kinds of stuff in the house. She kept us afloat for two months until we both got job offers. Jess has this determination to accomplish whatever she put her mind to.

All of a sudden, I had instant energy, and that little voice I always heard in the back of my head said, "Meditate." I didn't know anything about meditation. I always related it to yoga. So I started looking up YouTube videos on meditation. Once I found all the information I could find on meditation, I went on Amazon and ordered some soft music I could meditate to. I went back on YouTube and started looking at motivational videos. I made myself a video collection, like my Supermotivational Speeches, Day-to-Day Battles, Get Past Your Fears.

By this time, it was 2:00 a.m., and I really needed to get some sleep. Jess had just texted me that she had made it home safely. I made the mistake of texting her back right away, which led to her calling me upset because I was still up. I told her I was up doing some research and was waiting for her to text me that she made it home safely. She told me to get off the phone and get some sleep. I told her I loved her and for her to get some rest as well.

During the three to four weeks before my wife's next visit, I decided to start meditating before I went to bed. I was playing soft music while I slept, like soft jazz or classical. I would wake up with my pillow still soaked in sweat from dreams I didn't remember from the PTSD I was suffering from. I didn't let that stop me from my routine of early morning walking. I would walk all over the resort area for miles, looking up at the night sky. I remember walking down the main road of the resort area, making a left, and straight ahead I could hear the ocean.

It was unusually dark, but I knew at the end of the road there were two main resorts. The streetlights were lit on the main street but not on the street I was about to walk down. It was really weird because they were usually on. I started walking, and as I passed the third light pole, I stopped. I started to turn around because as a kid, growing up, I was afraid of pitch darkness. I would jump out of my bed on the top bunk and wake up my older brother to ask if I could sleep with him. He let me sleep with him anytime I was scared. But before I jumped in the bed, he would warn me, "Hey, you better not pee in my bed." I would jump in his bed first, then reply, "Okay, I won't," as I pulled the sheets up over my face.

So I was standing under this light pole, and that soft voice I heard in the back of my head said, "Look up." When I looked up—

wow. Scientists call it the Milky Way, but that night to me, it was God, the universe, something or somebody. When I looked up, I could see trillions upon trillions of stars. I could see them so clearly in all that darkness. I literally stood there for at least an hour, and I felt an overwhelming peace of mind. I started saying everything I was grateful for and thanked God for my beautiful wife's health and healing. I thanked him for my son's health and his new job. Then I closed my eyes and bowed my head. I thanked him for blessing me with the strength and knowledge to be a good husband, best friend, and caregiver to my wife, a good father and friend to my son. I finished my prayers with one simple phrase, "Thank you."

The most amazing thing happened. I heard this buzzing sound, but I couldn't tell where it was coming from. All of a sudden, the light I was standing under came on and was shining right on me. The lights in front of me started coming on, one after the other, all the way to where the sound of the ocean was coming from. I turned and looked behind me to see the first three lights were still not on. I started walking toward the resorts and the sound of the ocean. I made it to the last light. I turned around, and that was when the first three lights came on.

Now my basic human thought was to picture this guy in this electrical room realizing he forgot to turn on the lights to one of the main roads to the resort. But my feelings and my heart told me to look up and say thank you again. I looked up and, like a big kid, said, "THAT WAS AWESOME!" I looked around to make sure no one else was there.

The following weekend, my wife was flying in from Las Vegas for her second trip to the island. I was so excited to see her that I arrived at the airport two hours early and didn't care. When I finally spotted her in the baggage claim area, I grabbed her and picked her up. I didn't care who was looking. I asked her on the way to the car if she had dyed her hair. She said no. She noticed that her hair was growing back a little redder than it was before. She thought it could have been from all the chemo treatment or maybe it was just from walking in the sun a lot with Abby.

On the way to the resort, we were each filling the other in on what was going on. I told her about work, and she talked about packing up the house and having a yard sale. Once we got to the condo, I started telling her about all the research I was doing with meditation, motivation videos, and the law of attraction. She was so excited to hear everything, but she was even more excited to get a hold of one of those hamburgers. I started laughing as soon as she mentioned it because I was going to ask her if she wanted one. I was craving one as well. We drove over to the restaurant and got us some burgers and calamari to go.

After we finished eating, I started telling her about my routine with getting up in the morning and going for a long walk before work. It included listening to a couple of motivational videos every morning and meditating at night before bed. I also explained how I was studying the law of attraction and watching videos about that as well. A thought hit me right in the face as soon as I said law of attraction. I asked Jess, from the time she was diagnosed, and while she was going through chemo, what did she mostly think about? She said she was thinking about her healthy cells in her body and her liver healing. She told me she even looked at a picture of what a healthy liver looked like. She imagined her liver looking just like the picture.

Jess told me that she had deleted all the pictures from her phone that we took of her when her hair fell out. She even got rid of the pictures with scarves on her head. She said those pictures didn't look healthy to her. She asked me if I still had any pictures in my phone of her without her hair. I did have some pictures, but they were still there only to show me how far she had come in her healing. She asked me to please remove them from my phone because she wanted me to always picture her healthy.

I told her of course I would delete them and that I never thought of it that way. She said, "Subconsciously, a lot of people don't." I asked her if she realized she had been implementing the law of attraction in everything she was doing. She hadn't at first. She was just trying to keep herself in a positive frame of mind and steer herself away from a lot of negativity. I was excited because we both were doing the same thing, using the law of attraction. Sometimes, okay, probably all the time, Jess and I talk about so much stuff that we overlook talking about the little things. Like, "Hey, I'm watching videos on YouTube about motivation or the law of attraction."

We started sharing our videos with each other and still do it till this day. We both started to grow on the inside and outside because we were watching the videos so much. It was like we were reprogramming ourselves slowly from where we had been a year before that. Being on the island helped me because it was so relaxing and calming, except the day I went walking with my wife.

Jess would try to get me to go walking on my days off. The problem with that was that I was walking around at work all day in the sun. It wore me out. I felt bad when I told her no and reminded her why. So I decided to go walking with her. We, I mean my wife, decided to go on this long walk down the mile or so coast of the resort down past the beach. I was under the impression we were going for a short, easy walk. Once we made it to the beach, there were people everywhere. I was trying not to step on anyone that was laying out in the sun as we made our way through to the other side.

We approached a small hill that led to a cliff a little farther down the coast. Before we started walking up the hill, Jess turned around to ask me how I was doing. I assured her I was okay, and I actually was, until we started climbing that hill. As we climbed, we had to walk behind a lot of tall bushes and small trees. For some reason, it started to get hotter the longer we walked behind the tree line in between the bushes. I suggested to Jess, "Hey, let's walk out toward where we hear the water splashing." She agreed.

When we walked out from behind the bushes, *wow*, the view was amazing. The crystal-blue ocean water was hitting up against the rocks. It was something that you would see on a post card or a picture in one of those calendars. There were little holes in the rocks where the water would flow under and shoot out of the top side like a spout. I walked over to Jess and put my arm over her shoulder, and I pulled a Clark Griswold, you know, from the scene in *National Lampoon's Vacation*, when they were standing at the Grand Canyon and his wife asked, "Isn't it beautiful Clark?" As soon as Jess said, "Isn't it beautiful?", while moving my head up and down and tapping one foot, I said, "Yeah, it is. Okay, let's go." Jess started laughing because she remembered that movie scene as soon as I did it.

After that, we continued to walk down a little farther. I asked Jess if she wanted some water. I noticed that she was sweating, but I wasn't. She looked at me. "Hey, you're not sweating at all." She asked if I had been drinking water the whole time we were walking, which I was. She had a concerned look. "Okay, let's get you out of the sun for a while and then head back the condo."

As we walked back down the trail down the small hill, we both spotted a tree I could rest under right before we got to the beach area. We sat under the tree for about twenty minutes while I tried to drink as much water as I could. I told Jess, "As soon as I drink the water, my mouth gets instantly dry."

She declared, "You're definitely dehydrated right now."

I was like, "Look … you walked me into dehydration, woman." I started laughing. Jess didn't. She was worried, and I could see it in her face.

We started walking back to the condo. It was about two or three miles away. My wife was moving it. I was trying to keep up with her, but those little short legs were moving it. I think she realized, as she was speed walking to get me back and out of the sun, that she was making me dehydrate even more. She came back, apologized, and confessed that she was just trying to get me home. "I know, but I can't keep up with you today." We stopped at one of the neighboring resorts and sat in one of the covered cabana lounges along the walkway.

We rested there for a while when Jess said, "I know a shortcut to our part of the resort area." I asked her how she knew about the shortcut. She walked all over that area on each of her visits. I happily suggested, "Okay, let's do this, woman. Show me this shortcut you're talking about." We took all the shortcuts she knew, and next thing you know, we were back at the condo area in half the time. I was really impressed that she knew all those little shortcuts.

Once we got to the stairs to the condo, she had to help me up the four flights. I had completely lost all the strength in my legs and in my body. Jess was so worried and scared. I told her I would be okay. I just needed to rest and get some more fluids in my body. She laid me down on the bed. Even though I was dehydrated, I couldn't help but be amazed at my wife and how far she had come in her healing. I was so proud of her for keeping herself in such good shape and eating well while she was going through chemo.

The next couple of days I stayed in the condo, drinking plenty of fluids and trying to stay cool. Jess went out and picked up some groceries. During the afternoon, I had to make her get out of the house and go to the swimming pool. I told her I would be fine and that I could just lay down and rest while she was at the pool. She questioned me, "Are you sure, because I feel bad leaving you here."

"Woman, I am good. Plus I need to sit still anyway, so don't worry about me. You need to go and enjoy yourself."

Once I finally got her out of the condo, I started doing a search from my phone on waterfalls on the island and restaurants close to the ocean. I found the waterfall area, but not a good restaurant with a nice beach view. I rested for two days and told Jess I was going to take her somewhere special tomorrow. That morning we got up and went over to the resort gym located directly across the street from my condo. Afterward, we came back, took a shower, and ate some breakfast. I asked Jess if she was ready to go for a drive and see other parts of the island. She was so excited. "I am ready when you are!" We took off and headed for the waterfalls.

On the way there, I explained that I wanted it to be a surprise for her to see the waterfalls but didn't want to get us lost and take all day getting there. She agreed. "I don't want to get lost either, and I am excited to get there, so let me help with the directions." I told her if she could just keep a lookout for signs because sometimes they hid behind a lot of trees or those big colorful flowers that she liked. I was glad I did because we would have driven right past the turn we needed to take.

We had arrived at the waterfalls, and lucky for us, there were not a lot of people there. So we actually got to take plenty of pictures with the waterfalls in the background. After we walked around for a while, I asked Jess if she was getting hungry, because we had such a light breakfast that morning. She admitted she was getting a little hungry, so we set off to find a restaurant that sat right beside the ocean. It didn't take us long to find it, because I had made a wrong turn into this small hotel parking lot. Just so happened my wife noticed this restaurant sign that said, "Come and enjoy lunch or dinner on the beach."

I suggested, "Okay, do you want to try it?"

She said, "Sure, why not."

The place left me speechless. The people were nice, and the service was great. The food was excellent, and they had live music as well. Jess even pondered, "What are the odds of us taking a wrong turn and turning into this parking lot to find this place?"

I told her gratefully, "Today was a good day. We had a great workout, found the waterfalls, and found the restaurant we were looking for on the beach."

Well, it came time for me to take my wife to the airport the next day, but you know what, it wasn't as hard this time. Trust me, I was still going to miss her, but the sadness wasn't as bad because I knew I was going to see her in a couple of weeks. Plus, I knew she was going to be okay traveling back home in a healthy, safe, and relaxed manner. That was what my wife taught me while she was here with me. She told me to say that, picture her traveling back and forth in a healthy and relaxed manner, and that would calm me down, and it did. I kissed her and gave her a big hug, lifting her off the floor. I told her I loved her and would see her in three weeks.

I watched her until she made it through the metal detector, and then she disappeared. As I started to turn and leave, I saw this little hand wave out of the corner of my eye, and I turned and waved back. I knew it was her because she was jumping up and down, constantly waving. Plus, she called me, asking, "Did you see me waving?" She was out of breath, while we were talking, from all the jumping. She admitted, "Well, I wanted to make sure you saw my little hand because there was a lot of people around." I told her to have a safe flight, and she told me to get some sleep and don't wait up because "You have to work in the morning." I told her I would because I didn't want her to worry. She made me promise.

I started driving back to the resort area, and something told me to call my brother. Now normally my brother and I would call each other and talk about cars that we purchased or get caught up on family news. I could feel there was something, not necessarily wrong, but there was that voice in my head all the way from the airport to the condo constantly telling me to call him. As soon as I walked in the condo, I called him, and he actually picked up the phone on the first ring. You have to understand something about my brother. He's always working. On the off chance that he's not working, he's doing something like working on his motorcycles, his truck, or even the washing machine. But most importantly, taking care of his son, Markus.

You see, when Markus was born, he suffered from Group B Strep Disease, which caused him to have a fever as a newborn, in turn, caused him to have difficulty moving his joints. Markus cannot talk or walk, but he can still express himself through facial movement and sounds, especially when he is happy. My nephew had beaten all the odds from the time he was a newborn. The doctors would tell my brother and his wife that Markus would only live this long, or Markus would only live that long. Today my nephew is twenty-four years old and is very much loved each and every day by his dad, mom, two sisters, and the rest of our big family.

When my brother answered the phone, I knew instantly something was wrong because he didn't have that cheeriness in his voice. I asked him how he was doing. He said he was doing okay. I asked him what was wrong. He confessed, "I was just sitting here in the basement, thinking that I don't want Markus to pass away before me." When my brother said that, I could instantly feel his pain and sadness through the phone. I gathered my thoughts because it was time for me to be a big brother to my big brother.

I started off by asking how often he thought about this. He said, "Almost every day, really."

I asked him, "Is there something triggering it throughout his day?"

He replied, "We had a couple of close calls with Markus, and we had to rush him to the emergency room."

I asked him what type of close calls. He said one night Markus stopped breathing because he had fluid in his throat from when he was sick with a cold. My brother told me that he was always tired when all the negative emotions hit him. I said, "Okay, so what's happening is, the thoughts are coming into your head when you're tired. Then you replayed those episodes one after the other when you had to rush Markus to the emergency room."

He said, "I guess so. I never broke everything down like that."

I told him, "I did the same thing with Jess when she was diagnosed with stage 4 breast cancer. I was tired from not sleeping. I couldn't sleep because I was constantly worrying about whether she was going to make it through this or how long we had together. It was eating me up inside so much I was having nervous breakdowns all the time. I was having them in private, where no one could see or hear me, much like you're doing right now. The majority of the time, they took place in my closet because it was so easy for me to say I was cleaning my closet or getting rid of some old clothes."

My brother said, "I didn't know you were going through all of that. I knew you were going through some stuff but nothing that drastic. I figured you would have called me if you had gotten too bad."

I told him I had to work on the inside and the outside of myself so I could be strong enough to help and support Jess with what she was going through.

I assured him that he was stronger than he realized because he had been taking care of his son for twenty-four years. He gave Markus baths, fed him, picked him up out of his wheelchair, got him dressed, and put him to bed. He cut his hair, nails, and now shaved his beard. He took him on guy trips just two of them. I told my brother he was an amazing dad and caregiver. He had to believe that he was doing everything in his power to make sure that his son was going to live a good, loving, happy, and healthy life. I said, "You, your wife, and your two girls take such good care of your son. He is going to outlive all of us." My brother started laughing a little because he knew I was right.

I urged my brother to make sure that he was taking care of himself so he could continue to take care of Markus. I also told him he could start by finding some type of stress release for himself, "Like meditating or taking thirty-minute power naps when you know you're tired. You have to make yourself mentally aware when you're tired."

My brother thanked me and confessed, "I don't know how you knew to call me, but you called at just the right moment when I needed to talk to someone."

I didn't want to scare him about the voice that kept repeating for me to call him, so I just said, "Well, we haven't talked to each other in a while, so I decided to give you a call."

I told him one last thing before we hung up, "One day when I was visiting you guys, I was sitting in the living room watching a football game, and everyone was asleep. I walked back to check on Markus. You were sleeping across the room from Markus. Markus was about seven or eight years old, and I put my hand on his arm and said a prayer over him the same way our grandmother said prayers over us when we were little."

He said, surprised, "You did? I didn't know you did that. All these years … you never told me until now."

I replied proudly, "Hey, he's my nephew as well as your son."

"You are absolutely right," he agreed. Before we got off the phone, he told me he felt a lot better than he did before I called him.

I said, "Hey, that's what brothers are for, to watch each other's back and to support one another."

He added, "I think our grandmother and our mom were trying to teach us that when we were constantly fighting each other growing up."

"I was thinking the same thing."

Three weeks had gone by really fast, probably because of the fast pace of my work. It was time for my beautiful little wife to travel back over to the island of Kauai again. When she arrived, of course I had already placed an order for her favorite hamburger and cala-mari. She was so excited to see me! She ran over to me this time and gave me a big hug. It felt like I had just gotten off the plane and I was waiting for her to give me flowers and say, "Welcome to Kauai Island." I was like, "*Wow*, I missed you too baby. Was everything okay on the flight?"

She said enthusiastically, "Of course, I had a great flight and met some really nice people on the way over. Plus, I think we have the house sold as well because we have two offers. We were not getting any offers for a while, so I decided to use an affirmation that I had seen someone say on a YouTube video about selling their house." She could tell I was all ears to hear this.

She said, "Thank you, Lord, for the house selling so quickly" and "Thank you for sending us the right buyer for our home." She told me that was when the multiple buyers showed up two days later. Jess told me she started getting upset because she thought it was her fault that the house wasn't selling from the way she staged it. I told her, "No, I am pretty sure it wasn't that, because we bought the house, and it was empty." She said after she watched the video, she realized it wasn't her, and she just needed to wait for the right buyer to come along. Instead of one buyer, we got two. We made it back to the main road of the resort when Jess reminded me about picking up the food I had ordered.

After we got the bags in the door, we sat down and started eating. Neither one of us said anything for a while because the food was so good. I really didn't eat out a lot. I always liked saving that occasion for when my wife came over to visit me. I told her after I was finished with my food that I would like to take her to the beach on the navy base the next morning. She was really excited. I told her we could rent some water boards if she wanted to from the small recreational area. She was all for going to the beach.

The next morning after we finished breakfast, we headed out on our adventure. Once we arrived at the beach, we pulled into the parking lot. The beach was empty. It was so peaceful. I told her that everyone said it was going to be empty in the morning, but later in the day people would start coming out. She said this was a great idea. She loved that we had the whole beach to ourselves for a while. As we were walking to find a nice area to lay and put up the umbrella, Jess admitted, "I didn't realize when you said 'the whole beach' that we would have a mile or so of long beach to ourselves."

I said, "*Surprise!* You thought I was talking about a little small area of sand, like at the resort area, didn't you?"

"Of course I was."

After we found our little spot in all that sand, we decided to go for a short walk down the beach. I had to remind my wife, "Short walk, right? Not one of those walks like 'back to the coast of California' walks."

She started laughing. "No, not one of those 'I am trying to walk back to the States from here' walks." Jess tried to playfully push me and almost fell down. I caught her and stopped her from falling. I looked around to make sure no one else had arrived yet, and I grabbed her and put her in what I like to call "the couple playful headlock." It was not too tight, but it was not too loose either. Plus my wife had a little peanut head, so it didn't take much.

She was laughing the whole time. She was laughing so hard she made me start laughing. So I let her out of the headlock. I hugged her, told her that I was glad she was here, and I was missing her. She said she was missing me as well, and that was why she gave me such a big hug at the airport. I was like, "Oh, okay. I just thought you were sitting next to someone on the plane that was getting on your nerves so much that you were so relieved to see me."

She said, "No, actually, I had a very nice older lady sitting next to me. She was telling me about her family and why she was visiting Kauai." I told her I felt we were getting closer to the States with the walking and that we needed to turn back around. She teased, "Oh really," and started hitting on me. I started running. My body quickly reminded me that I was trying to run with flip-flops on very soft, thick sand.

Once Jess caught me, I was expecting her to hit me in the arm, so I braced for an arm shot. Little did I know, she was going to hit me in the right kidney area. As soon as she did, the whole right side of my body started tingling. It went numb, and I went down face-first into the sand like someone just shot my butt with a tranquilizer gun.

Jess ran past me laughing because she thought I was joking around. I think she forgot she had punched me like that years ago.

I was in the kitchen preparing my hot and spicy menudo. Jess was in the bedroom at that time, going through some old pictures she had found. I didn't want to interrupt her back-to-the-past moment, so I went to the kitchen looking for food. I found a can in the pantry of menudo I had hidden for emergency purposes such as this one. I started cooking, adding in some onions, lemon juice, and a little hot sauce for some extra spice. Next thing I knew, Jess emerged from the bedroom as I was doing multiple taste tests to get it just the way I liked it. She asked, "What is that nasty smell?"

"What nasty smell? I don't smell anything except for my delicious menudo."

She started sniffing all the way to me and said, "It's that menudo smelling like that."

I said "You mean this smell?" and then I blew my breath in her face.

Okay, first of all, I had never really seen my wife get really mad before, so this was new to me.

She said deeply, "Don't *ever* do that again with your breath in my face."

Of course, I started laughing and never really paid any attention to the serious look on her face, until it was too late. As soon as I blew my breath in her face for the second time, I felt this sharp daggerlike feeling in my lower right back. Jess walked off, and my right side started tingling. Next thing I knew, my entire right side went numb. I had a spoon in one hand and a towel in the other, and they both went straight up in the air. I thought about grabbing something to break my fall, but the only thing I could grab was my pot of hot menudo. First of all, I wasn't going to waste my menudo, and second, I wasn't going to get scalded by it either. I yelled "OH CRAP, WHAT THA —" and went down like a big buffalo in one of those old westerns, trying to make sense of what just happened.

Well, there I was, lying in the sand, and I knew what happened this time. My wife caught me again in the same spot. I laid there for a while. She came back over, still laughing of course. She asked me, "Are you okay? I didn't hit you that hard."

I replied, "I was expecting you to give me a punch in the arm, not another shot in the kidney."

"I'm sorry, baby." She helped me up, wiping the sand off me. "You always taught me to stick and move ..."

"Yeah, on someone else, not me. You're supposed to stay still and let me hit you back but in a soft, cuddly way."

Jess started laughing again.

As we walked back to our little area, we noticed the waves started getting bigger. More people started showing up. There was so much room on the beach that it still looked empty because everyone was so spread out in their own little areas. Jess and I decided to go out and try our little wave boards. The waves were too big, so we sat under the umbrella and started eating lunch, watching the waves come in. It was a really beautiful day out, and we just relaxed. We left the beach and turned in our water boards. I remembered that I wanted to show Jess the hand-carved tiki totems that this guy was selling on the side of the road across from the fish taco place I ate at sometimes.

When we pulled over on the side of the road and stepped out of the car, Jess smelled the fish tacos instantly as the aroma traveled with the breeze across the street. She asked, "What is that smell? It smells really good." I told her it was the fish tacos across the street. She was like, "*Wow*, all the food here smells really good. I'm sure they taste good as well."

I explained to her, "They're really good, and they're really large, plus you get two of them. I will go over in a few minutes to place an order. It will not take them long."

We started looking at the tiki carvings. There were so many of them my wife was going from one to the other. She would see one then find another one that was better than the next one. She was having another "Ooooo, somethin' shiny" moment. She would look and find another one. "Ooooo, somethin' shiny." At that time, we were both looking around, trying to find the one we liked the most. Then the guy laid a large turtle on the table, and my wife noticed it right away. It was too large not to notice, and the wood color on the back of the turtle was half dark wood, half light tan wood. My wife and I wanted the turtle for sure. I asked him if he could engrave our names on the bottom along with the date. "Sure, no problem."

I told Jess I was going to go across the street to order us some fish tacos. By the time I came back, she had picked out a wooden heart and had the guy to carve our first names and "Kauai 2015" under our names. I told her that was cool that she had found the heart amongst all the other tiki carvings. We both were getting hungry smelling those fish tacos. So I paid for both the turtle and the heart, and we headed back to the resort.

On our way back to the resort, Jess was holding the tacos. It was hard for her not to take a peek. I told her she could start eating hers if she wanted to but warned her, "If you start eating them, you won't be able to stop."

She said proudly, "No, I will wait until we get to the condo."

I looked over at her and teased, "Are you suuure you don't want to take a little bite?"

"Nope, I'm not gonna do it."

I teased her some more. "They're verrrry healthy, and they're made with purple cabbage and some island seasoning ..."

She caved in. "Okay, I will take one bite, and that's it." When she bit into that soft taco, she was like, "*Wow*, this is really good."

I bragged, "Told ya so ... all of the food is good at these little island restaurants."

We finally made it back to the condo. We ate the fish tacos on the balcony, watching the sun go down and all the lights at the resort coming on. It was really tranquil because some of the lights reflected off the water. We just sat quietly holding hands and listening to the local live music from the next resort over.

The next day, we just chilled out. Jess had to fly back the following day, and I wanted to make sure she was rested for her trip home.

I cooked her dinner that night, and we talked some more about what we wanted in our next new home. Jess told me she thought about her gourmet kitchen and decided she wanted two big islands, with enough space in between to walk through. I told her that would be great because she liked to make her own pasta. She also said she would like under-mounted lights in front of the islands. She described the floating cabinets in all the bathrooms with mounted lighting underneath them as well.

I told her proudly, "You really put some thought into all of this with the new house." She told me that she had a picture of everything in her head, and she was constantly adding to it. I told her she painted me a great picture of the house. I asked her how many garages she wanted. She turned around and asked me how many I wanted. "I was thinking of a three-car garage, and we can turn the third bay into a gym if you want." She said that would be awesome if we could do that. I said, "Of course we can, it's our house."

The next morning on the way to the airport, Jess told me she had found a rental house for us in El Paso. She said she thought she did good at finding this place because it was a three-bedroom, two-car-garage house.

She said, "The only problem is, it is a two-story, and I know you don't like stairs."

I assured her, "I don't have any room to complain about anything because I wasn't there to help you with any of it. I feel really bad about that, not being there to help you."

She said proudly, "I got this … I will take care of everything."

I asked Jess if she was nervous about her new job with helping manage such a large program and eventually taking it over. She was a little scared because she had never done that type of work before. She had always been in the field but never in an office. I assured her, "It's okay to be nervous because it's something new, but don't be nervous because you don't think you can do the job. You can do the job, Jess, you're really good at office work. Plus, you have good organizational skills, and you're very easy to get along with. You get to help people get jobs to support their families as well."

Jess said she hadn't thought of it like that. "Well, now I have a different outlook of the whole thing, helping people get jobs ... wow." This big smile came across her face. I knew I had found the magic word to get any doubt out of her mind, whether she could do the job or not.

We made it to the airport. I walked her to the baggage drop-off and then to the line for her terminal. We told each other we loved the other. I waited there until she made it through the metal detector. Then she jumped up and waved. I waved back. She disappeared into the terminal.

I started the drive back to the condo. I was thinking about her so much that a couple of times I looked over at the passenger seat to start a conversation. Then my phone rang. It was Jess calling me from the plane before it took off. She giggled. "You must have been talking because I could hear you up in my head."

I questioned, "Are you for real?"

"Yes, for real."

I told her that I was talking like she was there in the car with me. I was going over everything in my head we had talked about. "I looked over at the passenger seat to start having a conversation, but I forgot you were on the plane and not in the car with me."

She was like, "Awww baby, that's so cute."

I told her, "We don't use the word 'cute' in this family. I have been telling you that for the last nineteen years." She started laughing. "We use words like 'That is so awesome' or 'Cool' ... something like that. But never 'cute' in this family."

She said, "You're so cute still."

Then I started laughing and told her, "I love you, and try to get some sleep on the plane."

"Okay, I love you too," she said and then hung up.

Instead of me going straight up stairs to the condo, I went for a walk down to the beach. I figured if I was sad or upset and didn't know it, going to the beach and listening to the waves would calm everything down inside me. It worked because once I made it back up to the condo, I was able to meditate and picture Jess having a good trip back to Vegas in a healthy and relaxed manner. I was even able to sleep good that night as well. Jess had texted me to let me know she had made it safely back to Vegas.

Five days later, the house sold. Jess had already signed the lease for the house in El Paso. Our son helped the movers get everything out of the house in Vegas on time. Jess and Anthony Jr. both drove their cars to El Paso with Mia and Bear as passengers. Jess said they slept pretty much the whole way except when they stopped for a bathroom break or to eat.

They made it to El Paso thirteen hours later. The mover had gotten everything moved in really fast, and Jess had to start work the next day. Soon after my wife started working, my son had to start traveling again with his job. He worked for the same company we did but on a different program. I talked to Jess after her first day at work. She said they were throwing everything at her the first day, but it was okay because it helped the day go by quicker. She was able to have a little break after about four or five months and a little bit of traveling to Boston and California. She was able to come back over to the island of Kauai two more times and enjoy herself after some long workweeks.

Jess left Mia and Bear in good hands with a great dog sitter she had found in our local area. Out of Jess's last two trips over to Kauai, we were able to go to dinner at the restaurant a couple of times, ordering something different besides their famous hamburgers. We also managed to buy some more traditional tiki pole carvings. Jess was able to go shopping and find her shell necklaces she wanted. Soon after her last trip, my team and I were headed back to El Paso with our equipment. I couldn't wait to see my family, even though it had only been three weeks since I last saw my wife. I would always start missing her as soon as she boarded the plane from the island.

Jess was so worried when she picked me up that I wouldn't like the rental house. She was explaining about the stairs, how she couldn't find a house in a much better neighborhood within the budget we set. I leaned over and gave her a kiss on the cheek and told her I would like the rental house because she picked it out. I didn't have room to say anything because I wasn't there to help her. I told her if I did say something, she had my permission to give me one of her famous kidney shots. I started having a quick flashback of getting punched in the kitchen and on the beach. Which, by the way, was really embarrassing because when I had the slow-motion flashback, I realized there were people on the beach. To them, I probably looked like some big clumsy guy tripping in the sand. I quickly changed my comment to an arm punch, but a really hard arm punch. She started giggling. "No, I'm not going to punch you again."

I was like, "Really?"

She replied, "Really … and I didn't mean to punch you that hard."

She interrupted herself because she had realized she was supposed to go to the store after she had picked me up from the base. "I need to go to the store to pick up some things because I wanted to make you something special for dinner," she announced.

"Okay."

So we got to the store, and my wife wanted to examine everything on every shelf. Me, I was a typical guy. You give me a list of things to get, and I will grab everything on that list and be done. Okay, I might make one small detour to the chip aisle and then over to the frozen yogurt section, but that's it, no other detours and then I'm out. My wife wants to go full-on shopping again when she goes back in the store, even after she just went shopping the week before. When she does this, I just start giving her one of those very discreet man signals. "Hey, woman, I am ready to go." Jess would just look at me and smile with a little subtle giggle.

We finally made it up to the front counter. The lines were long. We made our way up to the cashier. She didn't look happy, because she gave me and my wife this tired zombie stare. Jess and I looked at each other, and I looked back at the cashier. "I know what you're thinking." She looked up and stopped scanning. I could see my wife looking at me in disbelief, and everyone behind us raised their heads up from looking at their cell phones. I said, "You're thinking that I'm the muscle, and she's the brains … Actually, I'm the brains, and she is the muscle," pointing at my wife. When I said that, everyone, including the cashier, looked at my wife and then looked at me and started laughing. While they were laughing, I continued, "Why do you think I'm standing here paying for the groceries and she's bagging them?" They started laughing more. Luckily the bags were not that heavy, or I would have bagged the groceries.

My wife was a way better organizer then I was. The only bagging rules I knew were do not put the eggs in with everything else, keep everything cold with the cold stuff, and do not crush the bread. I remember when I packed my suitcase for the first time around my wife. She asked me if I had everything packed, and of course, I told her yes. I didn't realize she had her way of packing, and I had my way of packing. My way was to pile everything on the bed, then separate it so I could take inventory of what I needed to pack and didn't need to pack. So far so good. Jess and I saw eye to eye on that part. That was when I saw my wife's skills at packing for the very first time.

I would fold my pants or roll them up. I would fold my shirts up as well, at least I thought I was folding them. When Jess opened my suitcase, it probably looked like a hot mess to her. It didn't make sense in her organized little mind. I could see the look on her face. I told her, "If you think you can do a better packing job than I can, then have at it." Then I walked out of the bedroom. I was probably gone for five minutes at the most. When I came back, my suitcase was organized like you would see in one of those hotel commercials when the person opened their luggage on the bed and the camera zoomed in on a perfectly packed suitcase.

I was so amazed that I was like, "What is this? How did you do this?" I couldn't stop staring at my suitcase. My wife took a mental inventory of everything I forgot. I pretty much forgot everything except for the main essential items. Well, let's just say it wasn't a good packing job on my part. My wife amazed me that day, and she had been amazing me for the twenty-two years I had known her.

As we walked out to the car, Jess said, "Only you could pull off something like that."

"Like what?"

She continued, "Make complete strangers laugh even if they're not in a good mood. Plus, you did it in a grocery line out of all places."

I asked her if she ever noticed when she was around unhappy, depressed, or just negative people in general how heavy the air or the atmosphere around her feels. She said, "I never thought about it, but now that you mention it, it did feel a lot better coming out of the grocery store for once." As we put the groceries in the car, I told Jess to hold that thought while I put the shopping cart in the rack. I got in the car, and we got out of the parking lot. I explained to her, "I think people go into the grocery store thinking about spending money. And they probably think about what they can afford and what they cannot afford to buy. I watch people's facial expressions more than I did before."

"Why more now?"

I continued on, "I think it developed from taking care of you."

She asked, "What do you mean from taking care of me?"

I told her that sometimes I would ask her how she was doing, and she would always say she was doing good. "I started watching your face when I asked you were you tired and you said, 'No, I'm not.' But your eyes said differently because of the gray around your eyes."

I told her I tricked her one day when I knew she was tired. I had her to come over and sit with me on the couch. I asked her if she was cold, and she had answered yes. I went in the bedroom and grabbed a small blanket and pillow. I told her to relax and I would rub her feet. She was so excited and grateful about getting the foot rub. As soon as I started rubbing her feet, she went right to sleep.

The funny thing about this was, I found this out years ago, that Jess whistled through her nose when she slept. This is so funny I have to tell you this story. It sounds like a little mouse is in the room. When I first heard it, we were in college at my apartment.

It woke me up out of a dead sleep. I thought there was a mouse in the room. I slid out of bed, trying not to wake up Jess. I grabbed one of my shoes and started crawling around on the floor, trying to find this mouse. I was looking under the bed and in the closet. Finally, I decided to stand still in the darkness to see if I could at least hear what direction it was coming from. I didn't hear it for a while until I started crawling back to the bed. I stopped. The mouse sound was coming from the bed. I was really upset then because the mouse had the nerve to crawl in the bed with us, wow. I crawled over to Jess's side of the bed because I could hear that I was getting closer to the mouse sound. I raised up next to Jess, and I could really hear the mouse then. I was on my knees with the shoe raised up in the air, ready to hit this mouse as soon as I pulled the sheets back. As I moved closer to Jess, I heard the mouse again. I moved even closer to Jess's face, thinking this mouse better not be sitting on my baby's face. I could see part of Jess's face and her nose. I put my ear close to her nose. I heard the mouse. It was Jess's nose! I fell to the side of the bed with my hand over my mouth, rolling around on the floor laughing and trying not to wake her.

Back to the car conversation.

I told her that day on the couch with her was when I started paying more attention to people's faces. She was like, "Oh, now it makes more sense."

Three months had passed, and my wife was really getting into her job. Her boss, Lenny, wanted her to travel to Boston with him to work on a contract proposal that had to do with the contract they were currently working on. Before she left for Boston, she was a little nervous about going. She felt like she wouldn't be able to add any input to anything because she was new. I told her that she would be fine, and she had the type of brain that absorbed information like a sponge. The information would come out when she needed it. I even gave her different examples of every time that had happened.

"Trust me, you will shine when the time comes." Jess smiled at me and said, "Thank you for always believing in me."

"We believe in each other."

"That's true," she agreed. She gave me a big, tight hug. I hugged the top of her head because she was so short.

I teased her, "Jess ..."

"What?"

"I can't breathe." We both started laughing, and she squeezed me even tighter. "Okay, I really can't breathe now." We both were still laughing as I tried to catch my breath.

While Jess was in Boston, she called me each night. We only talked for a short time because she was so tired from working such long hours. After the fifth day, she and Lenny had finished their part of the work on the proposals. They were heading back to El Paso the next day. When I picked her up at the airport, Lenny was waiting there with her to make sure she got home safely.

Lenny started telling me what a great job Jess had done in Boston on the proposals. He said that was the best time he ever had going up there to work on the proposals. My wife had this surprised look on her face as she smiled. I thanked Lenny for watching out for her and taking her to lunch and dinner with him. He said, "No problem." He had to get home to his family because they had plans for him as soon as he got off the plane. We both said bye and walked over to the short-term parking lot. Jess was holding on to my arm, happy to be home.

As soon as we got in the car, she started talking. It was like her brain was at a hundred miles per hour, and my brain was relaxed, cruising at around twenty-five miles per hour. I told her to hold on and let us get out of the parking lot first, then she could tell me everything. She was so excited, grabbing my arm, I started laughing. I will admit; I was just as excited as she was. I was just trying to get us out of the airport parking lot safely and onto Montana Avenue. It was a straight shot to our house on the eastside of El Paso. Once we got onto Airport Road, I told her to tell me everything.

She told me that everything happened the way I said it would. "My brain kicked in, and all this information came from out of nowhere. Once I started understanding everything, people started asking me for help. It was really great. Lenny was a great help, showing me everything and being very patient. I was surprised when he told you I did a great job because he just told me I was doing okay. He told you how good of a job I did. Maybe he was still in boss mode, and when we landed back here in El Paso, he went into relax mode. I guess that could have been it."

She kept going, telling me that she got to meet some really nice people there. She got to sit down and talk to her boss's boss. She told me that her next trip was coming up in three weeks to California and that it was mostly like a team building thing. Jess liked meeting people that she talked to on the phone and then being able to put the face with the name.

Jess got settled back into her work schedule after her trip to Boston. She called me from work one day and told me she was getting an achievement award. She said that Lenny was very happy with how she had performed in Boston during the proposals and had put her in for an award. She told me that it came from way out of left field and that she wasn't expecting that to happen. I told her, "You are very deserving of it, and you are capable of doing anything you want to do."

"I guess I am," she agreed.

Three weeks went by fast. Jess was on her way to California with some fellow coworkers, including Lenny and Lenny's boss, Charlie. Jess said once they got out to California, it was great, and everyone was enjoying the whole team building exercise. After Jess had returned home, she received a promotion to the next level up. She was on a roll and was doing really well in the office.

Jess didn't get a chance to have her breast surgery in Las Vegas and was still doing the maintenance treatments. She needed at least two to three weeks off from treatment before she could have the surgery. Selling the house, packing, moving, and me being in Kauai didn't allow time to schedule surgery. Dr. Malata had told Jess, before she left Las Vegas, it was okay to wait a little while longer because the lump in her breast was still shrinking.

Dr. Malata was really nice, and we missed her. She went out of her way to find Jess another cancer treatment doctor in El Paso that she would be comfortable with before she moved there. She also made sure that the new doctor, Dr. Amani, had all of my wife's medical and shot records. I told Jess that I would go with her on her next visit to meet with Dr. Amani so we both could talk to her about recommending a plastic surgeon.

We met with Dr. Amani a day before Jess's scheduled maintenance treatment. When she first walked in the room, I think she was a little taken aback because I was such a big guy. I guess it didn't help when I stood up and shook her hand. She was smaller than my wife. After she got over the initial shock of meeting me, we started talking about Jess having surgery soon to remove the lump from her breast. Dr. Amani asked to check the lump on my wife's breast. Jess told her it was still shrinking down because it was smaller than the last time she checked it. After she finished checking Jess's breast, she recommended us to Dr. Lauren. Dr. Amani informed us that Dr. Lauren was one of the top female reconstructive surgeons in El Paso. She scheduled us an appointment for the following Monday to meet with Dr. Lauren.

We met with Dr. Lauren that Monday. In the waiting area, there were pictures of Dr. Lauren's work on women who had reconstructive surgery. I was amazed that you couldn't even see the scars from the incisions. Jess walked back over from signing in at the front desk. She told me that from her doing research online that the scars would slowly fade. They wouldn't go away completely from what she gathered from looking at all the videos. By this time, one of the nurses called my wife's name. I didn't wait to be invited; I just walked back with her. I finally had come to the realization that the nurses and the doctor didn't care if I went to the back with my wife.

I noticed that other female patients didn't have partners with them. It was the same as in Vegas. Sometimes they would have their young kids with them or no one at all. Once we got to the back, the nurse weighed my wife and then checked her blood pressure. Afterward, she gave my wife an examination gown to put on and told us that Dr. Lauren would be in soon. As the nurse was walking out, Dr. Lauren was walking in the door with this big smile on her face. She looked like she had just stepped off a stage from doing a fitness model competition. I was waiting for her to say, "I am not a real doctor, but I did sleep at the Holiday Inn last night." But that didn't happen.

Dr. Lauren was really nice and very professional. I could tell that my wife wasn't just another patient to her. She told my wife that she went through her medical records and could see that she was taking care of herself. She said that her medical records showed that she didn't get sick from the chemo and that the spots in her liver disappeared and the lump in her breast was still shrinking. She said to Jess, "I see you did eight treatments instead of seven?"

"Yes, I did."

She asked my wife how she was feeling. Jess told her she felt great. The only thing that happened was her hair had fallen out, but it started growing back right away.

Dr. Lauren asked my wife if she could check her breast to see how large the mass was so she could get a good indication of what type of reconstruction she would have to do. Dr. Lauren was explaining to me and my wife as she checked Jess's breast that Dr. Kelvin would be working alongside her. He was the breast cancer surgeon, and they often worked together. She explained that he would go in and remove the mass and any lymph nodes that showed signs of still having cancer in them. Then she would come in and do the reconstructive part. We didn't know that; we thought she would do everything. She also explained, "It will probably be a three-hour long surgery because of all the nerves under your arm."

We were paying attention to every word and detail she was giving us. She grabbed a soft grease-like pen and showed us what the cuts would probably look like. Jess looked at me and asked me if I was okay. Then the doctor looked over at me. I told her I was okay and that I was really paying attention to everything. Jess smiled and said, "Okay, I just wanted to make sure you're okay with all of this."

I assured her, "I am good because I'm right here with you."

Dr. Lauren smiled at me and finished explaining everything. She told us she would make us an appointment to see Dr. Kelvin next week so he could go over his part of the surgery with us. We both said okay at the same time, and Dr. Lauren looked at us both. She said, "You guys are going to be okay."

The following week, we saw Dr. Kelvin. I would like to say this visit went as well as the one with Dr. Lauren, but it didn't. When we first met him, he must have been the only doctor there at the time because we were in the waiting room for about twenty to thirty minutes. Plus, when he first entered the room, my wife and I greeted him, and he said hello with no facial expression whatsoever. He asked my wife to put on an exam gown, and he would be back after she changed.

When he walked out the door, I told my wife, "There is something wrong with this guy, and if he thinks that I am going to let him cut on you with that nasty attitude, he better think twice." Jess was trying to calm me down the same time she was trying to get changed. She said, "It's okay, maybe he is having a bad day. Maybe the other doctors didn't show up or they showed up late." I told her that was no excuse for bringing his bad day in this room.

"When people come to see doctors, they're already scared or nervous. They probably already went through a lot or they wouldn't be coming here to have surgery. So he needs to take that into consideration as well."

She replied, "You're right, but let's just get through this appointment and we will talk to Dr. Lauren about this when we see her again."

"Okay, I promise I will not say anything to him."

A few minutes later, he knocked on the door and asked to come in. Jess answered him because she could tell I still wasn't happy with this guy. He came in and started checking my wife's breast and under her arm. While he was doing this, he explained about the lymph nodes and how he would have to remove all of them. I stopped him right there and questioned, "Remove all of them?"

He said, "Yes, all of them."

I replied, "Well, what if all of them don't show cancer?"

He said, "It's highly unlikely for one to have cancer and the others not to."

My wife jumped in because she could tell my questioning was starting to turn into an interrogation. She asked, "Is there a possibility that all the lymph nodes might not have cancer in them?"

He said, "Yes, about one in a million. You rarely see that in stage 4 cancer patients."

I finally broke my silence and said, "Well, there you go, Doc, there's the one in a million sitting in front of you."

My wife's eyes got big as to say, "I don't believe you just said that."

He wouldn't even look at me after my remarks and started explaining about my wife's arm staying swollen after the surgery and that was common. He said that it was because of the disruption of circulation from the removal of the lymph nodes. He also said that she would lose full range of motion in her arm. I think the thing that really made me upset was that he didn't say that there could be a possibility. Dr. Kelvin finished explaining everything. He told my wife she could get dressed and he would be back in a few minutes. I could tell he upset Jess a little about everything he was saying. I told her we would talk more once we got in the car.

Dr. Kelvin knocked on the door, and Jess told him to come in. He asked us if we had any more questions for him. We both asked him if we needed to set up another appointment with him before the actual surgery. He said yes and that we could talk to the receptionist on the way out. I told Jess to make the appointment after we saw Dr. Lauren first. I had a plan. Jess said, "Oh crap, a plan?"

"Yes, a plan. Trust me, it's going to work. So the next time we see him, he's going to be more positive, trust me."

Once we got in the car, I told her that we were going to get her in better shape. I explained further, "I mean better as in stretching more and doing more plyometric-type workouts. That will help with your healing and the flexibility of your arm."

Jess asked, "You thought all of this out while sitting in there?"

I said, "Yes, I did."

She asked, "What's the other plan?"

I told her, "When we go see Dr. Lauren again, we are both going to talk to her about Dr. Kelvin's bedside manner in general."

"Okay, but how is that going to change his attitude when we go back to see him next time?"

I told her, "Just wait and see."

The next time we had to go see Dr. Lauren, we told her about our visit with Dr. Kelvin. She was very disappointed because she spoke very highly of his bedside manner. She advised us to keep our appointment with him because the surgery was not that far away. Dr. Lauren gave Jess and myself the date for surgery. She asked Jess if it had been a while since she had maintenance treatment. It had been a month and a half, but she was still going in for blood work so they could make sure her numbers were good going into surgery.

The day came when we had to go see Dr. Kelvin again. Jess was so nervous about going to see him. "Don't be nervous. It's going to be all right, trust me." I put my hand on top of her hand as we drove to his office. She held on to my hand all the way to the office. Once we pulled into the parking lot, I told her to take a deep breath and relax. When we walked up to the receptionist desk, she told us to come around and that Dr. Kelvin was waiting for us. Jess squeezed my hand. I told her, "Step number two …" She looked at me. I looked back at her and smiled. The nurse showed us to the same room we were in before. She said Dr. Kelvin would be with us in a moment. We both said okay and thank you.

Jess asked me, "What is going on? It's different this time from the last time."

I asked her, "What do you mean?"

She said, "Everyone is really super nice this time. What do you think is going on, and what did you mean by step number two?"

I explained to her really quick before Dr. Kelvin walked in that talking to Dr. Lauren was step one. Walking in there, seeing a change was step two. Step three would be the change in Dr. Kelvin's attitude. Jess was like, "You're going to have to explain all of this after we leave here." I said okay.

Dr. Kelvin knocked on the door and asked to come in. Jess said to come in. Dr. Kelvin entered the room with this big smile on his face and said he really wanted to talk to us about our last visit. He asked my wife if she could please sit in the seat beside me while he sat in front of us. Dr. Kelvin started off by saying that he was very sorry for being so unprofessional and giving us a lot of the worst-case outcomes of the surgery. He said, "Mr. Randle, you were right … as far as we could see, from your wife scans, the cancer is in one lymph node. But we need to be absolutely sure once I start the surgery. I just wanted both of you to know that I am very sorry for the way I carried myself that day."

My wife replied, "I kind of figured you must have had a bad morning starting off."

Dr. Kelvin explained, "Yes, I was the only doctor that was here that morning, and there was supposed to be another doctor working as well. We knew that we were going to have a full schedule that day. But anyway, how are you guys doing?"

We told him that we were doing great and Jess was working with a personal trainer to get her body ready for the surgery, and it would help with her healing. She also told him that she had found this recipe to help keep her red blood cell count up before she went into surgery.

Dr. Kelvin said, "That is good. A lot of people don't think that far ahead like you guys do." He told us he had already talked to Dr. Lauren, and they had their game plan together for the surgery. He wanted to make sure that we knew the date was three weeks from this visit. We both told him that we did. His receptionist would have some instructions for us on the way out about what to do the night before surgery. Jess said okay, and we both said thank you.

After we got the instruction paperwork from the receptionist, Jess said, "Okay, now tell me, how did you figure all this out?" I told her it started with her. "It started with me?"

"Yes, you. I had a feeling you were right about Dr. Kelvin having a bad day. I did take that into consideration when we talked to Dr. Lauren about his bedside manner. Plus, she's older than him, and she spoke very highly of him. So for us to go back and tell her something different than what she told us about him was a little upsetting to her. I figured she was going to talk to him about us. I would understand if we went in his office in a negative mood and was rude to everyone, but we weren't. That's where I got the steps from. I envisioned our visit being much better than last time."

Jess said, "I did the same thing."

"You did?"

She said "Yes, I did" with excitement in her voice. "That is amazing, and I am sorry for earlier for being so nervous." I told her it was okay because she was the one having surgery. I was trying to get this taken care of because I didn't want anyone being upset and performing surgery on my wife. That was a no-no in my book. She said, "Thank you so much for taking care of me." We got in the car and gave each other a kiss. We headed back home because Jess had an early evening workout with her trainer.

As Jess got through all her workouts leading up to her surgery, I could tell she was going to be fine after the surgery. She was really pushing herself in the gym. During the morning of the surgery, I reminded Jess about not eating or drinking anything. Anthony Jr. and I were trying not to eat a whole lot in front of her. She told us to eat, and she would be okay. We still didn't eat a lot because we wanted to make sure we got to the hospital on time.

Once we got to the hospital, everything happened quickly. The nurse called Jess's name about ten minutes after we arrived, and away she went to the back to get prepped for surgery. Soon after, the nurse came and got me and my son so we could see Jess before she went into surgery. The anesthesiologist came in soon after we walked in and talked to all of us as a family. They started injecting my wife's IV with the anesthesia medicine. Afterward, the two nurses came over to take Jess off to surgery. I told my wife to tell some jokes in there up until she fell asleep. Everyone started laughing, including my son.

We walked back out to the waiting room, and soon after that, my son was headed for food. I knew it wouldn't take him long because he was a food connoisseur. Anytime he smelled food, he was heading in that direction. I remember when my wife made some of her homemade vodka sauce one night for dinner.

There was a lot of sauce leftover. It was late when we went to bed, so she left it in the big pot and was going to separate it in the morning to freeze it. That night I was awakened by a noise in the kitchen. I walked over to my bedroom door, cracked the door open, and looked around the corner to the kitchen. My son had the pot, I mean the whole pot, up in the air, drinking it like it was water. I couldn't believe my eyes. I said, "Hey, what are you doing?"

He was like, "What? I don't know what you're talking about. I was just standing here, admiring this delicious sauce Jess had made."

I started laughing, and so did he with sauce all around his mouth. I told him Jess was going to kick his butt for drinking all her pasta sauce. I told him to put the rest of it back and go to bed. He was like, "Okay, Pops." He got his appetite honestly from me, I guess, because his uncle and I would eat like that, and we were smaller than my son.

When my son came back after being gone an hour, it looked like he brought back groceries. It literally looked like a small bag of groceries, but it was probably a snack for him. I said, "Son, did you leave any food in the cafeteria for the people that actually work in the hospital?"

He said "Of course I did, Pops" and started laughing.

I told him, "They probably wanted to tell you as soon as they saw you, 'You do know this is not a buffet, right?'"

We both started laughing because he knew I was right. I was really glad he was there with me. The time went by fast because we were talking about cars and jobs and his future in contracting.

Soon after, the nurse called out, "THE RANDLE FAMILY." I waved in her direction. We both jumped up and met the nurse at the door. She said that Jess was doing good, and she did really well in surgery. The nurse was explaining to us that Jess was still a little groggy from the anesthesia, so she might be in and out a little. She had drain tubes under her arm as well from the extra fluid draining. We made it back to the recovery area, and she was awake and smiling. We both stood on each side of her. I grabbed her hand and asked her how she was doing. She said she was doing good but could tell they did a lot of cutting on her because she could feel all the bandages on her. Dr. Lauren and Dr. Kelvin decided to keep my wife there overnight to make sure everything was okay with her.

She started healing really fast after leaving the hospital. Within two weeks, Dr. Kelvin had removed her drain tubes from under her arm. He told us that we were right; only one lymph node had cancer in it. It was incredible that the cancer stayed in that one area. We both looked at each other and smiled. Dr. Kelvin noticed that my wife's arm wasn't permanently swollen and that she almost had full range of motion. He couldn't believe everything he was seeing. He said, "Whatever it is you guys are doing, keep it up."

We said, "We will, and it's all part of our lifestyle change."

He asked, "Lifestyle change?"

My wife explained, "Yes, we decided we were not going to call it a diet or change of routine or anything like that. We decided to say we were making a lifestyle change for our health and everything we do in our life from here on out."

We could tell he was a little blown away because he probably never met anyone like us before. The next day we had our appointment to see Dr. Lauren. She told Jess she could return to work, but she had restrictions not to lift anything heavy, over ten pounds, for another two to three weeks. She also explained to us she wanted to wait awhile and give Jess the choice of when she wanted her to perform the second surgery to fully complete her breast reconstruction. Jess told her she would wait a couple of months because that was a big surgery in itself. Dr. Lauren agreed and fully understood about Jess needing a break from the surgeries.

My wife returned to work like she never missed a day. Her bosses had called me during her surgery to make sure she was doing okay. They were happy to have her back as well because she was a significant part of their team now.

Jess and I had talked about going out, looking at a lot of the open houses that were taking place on the weekend. One day after work, she was on the computer, looking at different websites on houses for sale. She had come across this house that really stood out to her. She told me I really needed to look at this house. I ran over to the computer, and I was amazed myself at the house. The thing that started everything in motion with this house was the kitchen itself.

When my wife was scrolling through the pictures of the house, she stopped on the kitchen picture and said, "That's my kitchen."

I looked at her. "Your kitchen?"

She said, "No, no, I mean, that's the kitchen that's been in my head this whole time. Look at the picture … you see the large split island, the modern air vent over the stove, the pot filler over the stove? Look at the backsplash on the walls. That's my modern kitchen right there. I can't believe this house has all my ideas that I want in a house. Look, they're having an open house all this weekend."

I told her, "Let's go over tomorrow and check it out."

"For real, you really want to go over?"

I said, "Yes. Anytime you're super excited about something like this, then we need to check it out."

She said "Thank you, thank you so much" and jumped up from her seat and into my arms. I picked her up and walked back to the kitchen with her in my arms and sat her on the counter while I finished cooking dinner.

That morning, Jess was so excited she was up like she was going to work. She had fed Mia and Bear already, ate something herself, and had made me and Anthony Jr. breakfast. I woke up to the smell of bacon, and my son was still asleep. I got dressed. I had just remembered we were going to go see the house. I ran downstairs, kissed Jess, and started playing with Mia and Bear. Then sat down and started eating my breakfast. Jess asked me "Are you excited this morning!" like she just drank some high-quality H_2O pot of coffee.

I was like, "Yes, I'm really excited, but I can tell you're super excited."

"Yes, I am!"

I told her, "Okay, we have to go in there with a plan. We can't just run in there and say we like your house, we want to buy it now. We have to go in there calm, cool, and collected. Make sure we ask plenty of questions about the house and the builder."

She said with a lot of excitement in here voice, "Okay! Okay!"

I said, "That doesn't really sound like calm, cool, and collected to me. That sounds like you're on the verge of breaking out in a happy dance as soon as we get there, woman."

She said, "No, I am just super excited, but when I get there, I will calm down."

"Okay, you sure?"

She said "I'm sure" with a big smile on her face.

We drove over to the west side of El Paso over Transmountain. As soon as we got over the mountain, it reminded us of parts of Las Vegas somehow. We felt a sense of comfort and peace as soon as we got over the mountain. It felt like home. As we pulled up in front of the house, we were both excited. We had to calm ourselves down. We walked in the house, and the Realtor had this big smile on her face. She told us to come on in, and she introduced herself. "Hi, my name is Franki, and welcome to our open house today." Franki was really nice and down to earth and was dressed very professionally. She had a very calming personality about her. She told us to walk around and if we had any questions to feel free to ask.

As we walked around over toward the smaller bedrooms, we noticed the color pattern of the interior right away. It was a steel gray with a tint of blue in it, which we liked. The bedrooms were small because the builder had installed a loft in each of the bedrooms for kids. The stairs took up some of the square footage in the rooms. Those rooms would be fun for kids because the loft had a nice railing around it. You could see kids up there playing like they were flying a plane or a spaceship from up there. I told Jess, "Let's walk over to the garage and then we can go to the master bedroom."

"Okay."

We headed to the garage, and Franki walked to the garage with us. As soon as I saw the garage and the painted floor, Franki had me at hello. I know what you're thinking. Typical guy, but not necessarily. Give me a chance here. The garage floor was painted gray with the colored small spots on it, which I liked. It also had the small energy-efficient tankless water heater that my wife and I wanted. There was something else in the wall close to the garage door that was covered with Plexiglas.

As I walked over to it, Franki started explaining, "The glass is covering the spray foam that we use throughout the house."

Jess and I lost our composure and turned to Franki and said, "You guys use spray foam throughout the entire house?"

Franki said, "Yes, the builder foams the house from top to bottom at no additional cost to you."

Okay, right there was where I almost lost it again. Jess was on the verge of breaking into her happy dance. I asked Franki, "Could we take a look at the master bedroom and master bath?"

She said, "Sure. I'll let you guys go in, and I will be there soon because I think I hear someone else out here."

We both said okay.

As we walked through the kitchen, there was another couple that had just walked in, and Franki went over to greet them. When Jess and I walked in the room and looked up at the ceiling, "Wow" was all I could say. My wife, on the other hand, turned to me and said, "I think two drops of pee just came out." I told her that was nasty, and she could have said "I soiled my pants" or something. She said it wouldn't have been as funny. I told her that was funny because I wasn't expecting her to say that.

As I walked around the bedroom, taking inventory of what I liked, Jess walked into the master bath and said, "You need to come in here, like right now." When I walked into the master bathroom, I instantly felt like I was in a high-end spa. The shower was located right in the center of the bathroom, and it was encased in thick glass with smooth river rocks on the shower floor. It also had a big rain showerhead on the ceiling and showerhead on the wall. I told my wife these were all the things that we saw on the house channel. She said, "Where did you think I got all of my ideas from?"

"I thought maybe you were taking in a lot of that stuff you were seeing on the house channel."

She said, "You have no idea ..."

After we walked out of the master bath, we stopped and looked inside both his and her closets. Jess said those were the custom closets she had wanted in our house in Las Vegas. There was a swirl design built out on the ceiling. I told Jess, "I would like to have that ceiling in our master bedroom, but I would like it painted different so it can stand out." She agreed.

We walked into the kitchen, where we met Franki. She asked if we wanted to see the size of the backyard. "Yes, please." It was a really nice backyard, too small for us, but we liked the way it was designed. She asked us how we liked the house overall. We told her we really liked it a lot because it was modern and different. She asked us if we were preapproved already. I told her that we were. She said, "Great! Would you like to put an offer in?" I was like, "No." We said we liked the house, but I didn't want to put in an offer. By the look on her face, I think she realized at that moment this wasn't our first time buying a house. I could tell she was trying to recoup herself, and she did.

She said, "Well, we do build houses to any floor plan you want."

My wife said, "Really?" and that was when Franki knew she had us back again.

She said, "Oh yes. The builders are great people, and they will work hand in hand with you, every step of the way, with the building process. Would you like to meet the builders tomorrow?" We both hesitated a little and Franki said, "Trust me, you're going to like them."

We both said, "Okay, we will come back tomorrow around the same time."

The next day we went back. Franki was standing in the kitchen with the builders, Dean and Ann. Dean introduced himself and then introduced his wife, Ann. They both were very nice, but we could tell that Dean was the closer of the group. He asked us what we were looking for in a house and asked us to "take this house, for instance."

My wife said, "The Jetson house ..."

Everyone turned and looked at my wife. Dean said, "What did you call this house?"

My wife explained, "I named this house the Jetson house because it looks super modern on the outside."

Dean said, "I never thought of it like that ... the Jetson house ... Okay, the Jetson house it is."

"So what do you like and what do you not like about the Jetson house?"

I looked at my wife because I knew she had this photographic memory with this filing system in her head of what she liked and didn't like. I told Dean, "Why don't you walk around with my wife and she will go down the list of things. Plus, she's going to tell you everything that's wrong with this house, building wise."

Dean looked at me, looked at my wife, and said, "Okay, Mrs. Randle, let's go." He asked Jess where she wanted to start. She said, "Let's go through the small bedrooms first and then over to the master bedroom." He looked at me, Franki, and his wife, Ann, in disbelief, like "Wow."

I sat and talked with Ann and Franki and explained to them that my wife already had the house up in her head she wanted built. They were like, "Okay then."

Ann asked me, "Does she know what color she wants the interior and exterior?" I told her yes, and then Ann said, "Wow, you guys are going to make this easy."

Franki asked me, "Does she know what she wants her kitchen to look like?"

I said, "Yes, we're actually standing in it."

She said, "Are you being serious right now?"

"Yes, I am. This is the kitchen my wife always wanted."

Ann was so proud because she had put the kitchen together herself with all the color combinations, appliances, and the cabinets.

I told them that we had been looking for a house for a year now but never could find anything we really liked. I said that my wife and I decided we needed to build a home with everything we wanted in it. Jess and Dean had finished walking around the house. Dean said, "We need to get the workers back over here because Jessica found some measurements that were way off in the closets. Also, when we went outside, I noticed we needed to put a drain in as well." Dean looked at Jess and said, "I need to hire you."

Dean and Ann started talking to us about the different model houses they had, and nothing really spoke to us on the house plans they had. We asked them if we could design our own house plans. They told us that they had someone that would sit down with us and help us draw out the house plan for us. I was thinking to myself, *Okay, this conversation just got interesting.* They asked us if we were ready to commit to signing with them on getting a house built. We asked them if they had a couple of large lots we could choose from.

"There are still a couple of large lots left. Would you guys like to go over and pick your first lot out and then we're going to have you pick a second one as well. Sometimes the developer will sell a lot and forget to post it, so we like for our clients to pick two, just in case one of the lots is sold already."

We picked out our first lot, and then we picked out the second lot, which happened to be right beside our first choice. After we picked out the lots, we went back to the Jetson house, signed our agreement, and put down a deposit for the land.

On the drive back to the east side, we were so excited. We were screaming in the car and laughing. The next day, which was a Monday, Jess got a call at work from Ann. She said, "I have some bad news, and I have some good news. The bad news is the first lot you guys picked out was sold, but the second lot is still available."

Jess said, "That wasn't really bad news because we still get to build our house on a lot we picked out."

Ann said, "You're exactly right. Well, congratulations on the start of your new home!"

Jess said, "Thank you, thank you, thank you very much!"

Ann and their architect wanted to meet with us that week to draw out some plans for our new home. Jess was like "Really?"

Ann said, "Yes, we don't mess around because we have to get permits and everything. It takes a while to get permits approved here in El Paso."

Jess told Ann we could meet her on Friday because she had a short day on Friday. Jess called me with so much excitement in her voice. She told me about the appointment on Friday, and I told her I had just gotten off the phone with our mortgage guy, Zach. Zach said our approval letter was still good for another four months, so we were good. It was great that everything was moving the way it was moving. Jess said she had something to show me when she got home from work.

When Jess got home, she asked me to come upstairs for a minute. She had me close the door because she wanted to show me something. She went in her closet and pulled out this box she had made. Inside the box were pictures of appliances, countertops, lights, modern fireplaces, furniture, everything that would make up a house. She even had a stainless steel big refrigerator freezer combo that we had always wanted in our house. I told her I would love to have that big refrigerator, but those normally ran between $5,000 to $15,000 depending on what brand you bought. She said, "Well, if it's in my vision box, we're going to get it and put it in the house."

By the way, this was my wife's vision box. It had white paper wrapped around it with stars and glitter on it. I told her okay, because I had forgotten for a brief second who I was talking to. "I believe everything in your vision box will be put into our new home. Where there is a will, there is a way."

She said, "Exactly. Don't worry about the price of everything. I believe everything will be made affordable to us somehow. Plus, I am going to keep a budget of everything as well."

Friday came, and we were sitting down, meeting with Dean, Ann, Franki, and Nancy, their architect. We started off talking about square footage and then the number of bedrooms and the number of garages we wanted. Jess said she wanted a large laundry room with a doggy shower in the laundry room with an area for Mia and Bear to sleep. Something like two cubby holes so we could put their pillows in for them to sleep on. Also, we wanted to have their doggy door in the laundry room as well. Everyone but me was looking at Jess like, "Wow, she really knows what she wants in this house."

She had the measurements for all the bedrooms, the kitchen, the master bedroom, and the bathroom. Dean and Ann asked her what she wanted her master bathroom to look like. She turned to me, and so did everyone else. I told you I wasn't just your typical guy when I was looking at the garage. I told them, "We would like a spa-like master bathroom. I would like a XL tub straight ahead when you first walk in the bathroom. A wall in between the tub and the shower with a large glass window between them. Also, we would like a large rain showerhead above us and then a regular showerhead on the wall as well."

Ann said, "What do you want as far as cabinets and countertops?"

That was when Jess stepped back in and said, "We both would like floating cabinets with lights underneath and countertops using the same material and color that's in the kitchen."

Before we left that night, we had completed the whole house in a couple of hours.

Nancy said it would take her a couple of days to put everything together, and she would give us the complete drawings with the electrical and plumbing. Within a couple of days, like Nancy said, we had the drawings. I told Jess, "This is out of your little head, your house."

She replied, "No, our house."

We were looking over the plans, and we just added some more wall sockets and added two more camera outlets to the outside wall. That was it. Once we sent the plans back to Dean and Ann, they had to submit them for approval to the City of El Paso.

It took about two weeks to get the approval, and once that happened four days later, Dean started on the foundation. We did a walk-through with Dean and Ann once they had the outline down of the house. I was looking around and asked Dean, "Are you sure you have the square footage right, because this looks smaller? Our three-car garage looks like a two-car garage, and it doesn't look like there's enough room to pull the car into the driveway because of the wall."

Dean said calmly, "No, it's the right size. It always looks like it's not that big until we pour the foundation, and then you can see the actual size."

I looked at Dean. "You probably get this response a lot when you lay the outline down for building your houses?"

He said, "Yes, I do, but some are worse than others. Some people will actually bring their own tape measure and measure it with me."

I said, "Okay, that's a little extreme and unnecessary."

Dean just smiled and continued explaining the different steps with laying the foundation and the framing of the house.

Ann and Jess were walking around, talking about the colors of the interior and exterior of the house. They were also looking at the backyard and discussing about removing a lot of the dirt from the back upper part of the developers' walls so we could have more yard. Dean looked at the backyard and said, "That can be done because we were going to put you guys another retainer wall up for your house as well." Dean told us that in the next two or three days, they were going to start pouring the concrete for the foundation. Ann told us everything moved pretty quickly up until we started doing the walls and then it started to slow down. We asked them both, "How long will it take to finish the house?"

They said, "Normally six months, but we wanted to ask you guys if we can take seven months so we can come in, test everything, and fix anything we might have missed. Plus, that will give the house enough time to settle as well."

We were like, "Okay, that would be no problem."

A couple of days later, they started laying the foundation, and it was really cool to see. I wasn't able to be there because I had just started a new job in lower east Texas, so Jess had to send me pictures. A week or two later, they started putting the frame up and running the electrical wiring through the house.

Later that week, I received a call from Jess. She told me she had just gotten back from one of her checkups, and she was back at work, sitting in her office. She told me that the doctor had looked over her scans and found a spot on her ovaries. She said that a lot of women had these little cysts on their ovaries. It was just with hers they found some little lumps on top of the cyst. The doctor told her that since she had stage 4 breast cancer, they didn't want to take a chance and leave it in there. They thought it would be best to have her ovary removed. I asked her when they wanted to do the surgery; she said as soon as we could schedule it.

I told her, "Okay, I just need to clear it with my boss because I just started two weeks ago, so I don't have any time saved up." I called my boss and explained everything to him, and I could tell with the words he was using that the answer was going to be no. He told me I couldn't leave because I was the site lead, and it wouldn't look good on the company if I just got here and then had to leave. I told him I understood, but really, I didn't, at least not in my heart anyway.

I called my wife back and told her I wouldn't be able to make it because of the job. She said it was okay. I told her it wasn't okay because I needed to be there for her. She said, "Well, the good thing is Anthony Jr. is here, so I won't be alone." I told Jess I had completely forgot he was there because he traveled so much. I told her to let me speak to him.

I told my son, "Pay close attention to what the doctor says both before and after the surgery because sometimes Jess doesn't absorb everything the doctor tells her after the surgery. Have her there a little early, just like we did last time."

He told me, "Okay, Pops, I got this."

"I know you do, and I have complete confidence in you."

I talked to Jess a little while longer, and then I called the builders and our Realtor, Franki, and explained everything to them, including me not being able to come home for a while. I asked all of them if they could help my wife as much as they could through the building process of the house. They all said that would not be a problem, and they asked what hospital she would be in. I was very grateful for all of them, including Franki, because she would always show up early and always wanted to be there to look at everything with us. She even went out of her way to show us some more houses that Dean and Ann had built so we could get some more ideas for our house. I think she showed us about five or six houses, and each one of them had something in it that we liked. Franki was a great Realtor in my book. Like I said before, she had me at hello, because she was very professional.

Anthony Jr. kept texting so I wouldn't worry so much. I told him he did not have to text me so much because I knew he was there with his stepmom. I told him to tell her to call me before she went into surgery and then for him to call me when she came out of surgery. I talked to her just before she went in. I told her I loved her, and she would be in and out in no time. She said "I love you too, baby" and that she would talk to me after the surgery.

Ann and Dean were moving along on our house and making great progress. The foundation was laid, the frame of the house was up, and the electrical and plumbing were installed. They started doing the roof and the sheet rock, and then it all started to come together. They started on another house, so Jess could have time to heal so she could look at everything before they started spraying the foam insulation.

Meanwhile, Jess was doing great after surgery. She was healing up at her normal quick pace and was back at work within seven days after surgery. She was so excited to go over to see the progress on our house. After she and Dean walked through to look at all the progress, Dean scheduled the guys to start spraying foam in two days. That also gave me enough time to fly in to see them start spraying the house.

When I landed in El Paso, I was so glad to be home and to see my family. Jess was waiting for me at the airport, and my son was at work on the nearby base. As soon as I saw Jess, I gave her a big hug and told her that I missed her so much. She had missed me very much as well. After I got my bag, we headed out the parking lot, and we were off to the west side. I told Jess, "No matter how many times we drive over this mountain, it always feels like home over here on this side."

"Yeah, I feel the same way every time I drive over here to check on the progress of our house."

As we pulled up to our house, Franki, Ann, and Dean were standing out front. The guys were dragging the equipment from their van to the house to start spraying foam on the inside of our house. Once they got their equipment set up and their suits on, they started spraying the garage. Dean stopped for a minute to show us how the foam crawled into any open cracks that might not be sealed. It was our first time having foam insulation sprayed in our home, so it was very interesting to see. Soon after the guys started spraying, our son drove up to the front of our house. Dean told him he could go watch them spray the foam in the garage. He thought it was the coolest thing to see.

Ann and Dean were on schedule with everything. Dean asked Jess if she wanted anything different in the house that she might have forgotten to bring up during our discussion of our house plans. She said, "Yes, there was one or two items I forgot to tell you about. I will send you pictures and measurements later tonight or tomorrow morning."

Dean said "Okay, not a problem" and asked if we wanted to take a tour through the other houses they were working on. My son said yes and started walking off really fast, had no clue where he was going, and everyone started laughing.

We went and toured about three houses that they were working on in the general area. The third night I was at home, I was having trouble sleeping. I was trying not to wake my wife up, but she was already awake. She asked me if I was having a bad dream or something. I told her, "No, I think I am a little upset because I have to leave on Tuesday. Plus, I am excited about our house as well." She told me she wasn't really sleeping well either, and that was probably what was keeping her awake, me leaving and the excitement of our house. I suggested, "Since we both really aren't that sleepy, let's go for a drive and look at our house again."

"Are you sure? It's three thirty in the morning."

I said, "Sure, because it's going to take us a while to get dressed, and I need to let Mia and Bear outside for a while. Then we can take our time driving over to our new house."

Once we finally left the rental house and took our time driving over, it was around 4:45 a.m. when we arrived over Transmountain. We pulled right in front of our new house as the sun was starting to come up. We walked along the outside of the frame to the backyard. Then we walked inside. It was amazing. We could finally start to see our house and Jess's picture that was in her head all along. Jess started taking me for a tour in the master bedroom.

She asked me, "I bet you can't guess what this is?" There was a three-fourth wall that was bumped out from the full wall, and it ran straight up to the ceiling. I told her I didn't know, but it looked really familiar, like I saw it somewhere before. She said, "You did. It's in my box. You remember, with the glass fireplace with the different-colored flames."

I let out this big yell, "ARE YOU KIDDING ME! The fire place we always see on the house design channel?"

"Yes, and there will be rope lights running all the way around behind the bump out part."

All I could say was, "Wow, Jess I wasn't expecting this. You're amazing."

As we walked in the master bathroom, it looked small. I guess I had this look on my face because Jess caught it quick. She asked, "What's wrong?" I told her I thought the bathroom looked a little small. It didn't look like there was enough room in there. She reassured me it was, and it just looked that way because it was an empty space right now. We walked out to the kitchen, dining, and living room area. Jess started explaining where everything was going to go. She had this mental picture of everything. I told her I was sorry I couldn't see everything that she could see when it was a blank canvas to me. She walked over and rubbed my back. "That's why I am here explaining everything … so you can see it."

We walked around the house a little bit more. When we walked out to the car, we turned around to take a look at the house again. I grabbed Jess close to me and told her I loved her, that I was very proud of her and very grateful for her. She said, "Thank you, and I'm very grateful for you too for being so patient with me and my ideas for the house."

I told her, "Stop it … You had me at hello." She started giggling.

Tuesday morning came, and I was at the airport. Jess had an early meeting, so she had to drop me off and get everything prepared. About three weeks had gone by, and during that time, Jess had been sending me pictures of our house. When she couldn't make it over to take pictures of the progress, Franki would go over and take pictures. If Franki or Jess couldn't make it over to see our house, Dean and Ann would take pictures (with Dean posing in the picture and making faces). It felt like Jess and I got the better deal with building this house. Like I said before, a great Realtor and great builders.

During this time as well, my son was back overseas with a company working on UAVs, which he loved. It was something different and new that he enjoyed. Me, I was glad to be doing contract work in the States. I was heading to El Paso to see my beautiful wife and our other two kids, Mia and Bear, and our new house. Jess had picked me up from the airport late, but I didn't mind at all. I knew she was having late meetings all during the week. Plus, she had grabbed some food for us both on the way to the airport. She asked me if I wanted to go over to see our house, and I said, "Yes, of course."

"Good, because we are going that way anyway." We both started laughing.

On the way over, she told me she had a couple of surprises for me in our house. I said, "A couple of surprises for me, really? You know I don't like surprises, so tell me, what is it?"

Jess said, "You will have to wait until we get to the house, but I just know you're going to love them."

When we arrived at the house, the exterior paint and the stucco were finished. The exterior paint was the same color gray that was on the Jetson house, which she knew I liked.

She told me she had an idea for the stone color she wanted on the house. She asked if I would be willing to run around with her tomorrow to find the stone. I told her yes, as long as she had some places already picked out we could go to. Jess told me that Ann had given her the address to three good places we could check out. I told Jess if she could be the navigator, I would drive us around tomorrow. "Okay, it's a deal."

When we got to our house, we walked in, and it was great. They had laid the floors down. The split islands were in the kitchen along with the countertops and cabinets. Dean was there and said to me, "I have something over here for you."

Jess said, "It's one of your surprises!"

They had found me an XL tub! I was like, "Where did you guys find this tub?"

Dean explained that they had to order one for another client that had bought a house on the east side, and this guy was six feet, six inches. Our tub was sitting in the dining room area when everyone told me to get in to see if I fit. When I stepped into the jetted tub, I felt like a little kid in this huge tub—it was awesome.

Jess said, "I have something else to show you. Follow me into the master bedroom. Look up."

I was like, "Wow, look at the ceiling." It was one of those ceilings you could wake up to every morning and lay in bed just staring at it.

She said, "Now look at this …" It was the bump out wall idea she had described to me with the glass fireplace. It was in our bedroom with LED lights behind it. I am not going to sit here and lie to you. I was blown away with everything that my wife had put into the house.

Dean told me that people would walk through our house, asking him if it was for sale. Ann said, "Just last week we had three families walk through, and all three of them wanted to buy your house."

Jess said, "Wow, so I guess I really did do a good job with our house."

Everyone said, "Yes, you did, you did a great job with everything you picked out."

After I looked at everything in the master bedroom, we walked into the master bathroom, and my wife said, "Watch this." She turned off the lights. She turned on another switch, and the light came on under the cabinets. I said, "Floating cabinets with LED light! We wanted something like this for a long time and now we got it!"

Jess said, "And now we got it."

Everyone around us was all smiles. Ann said, "You guys have an appointment to pick out your appliances tomorrow."

Jess said, "We were going to go to the stone places tomorrow."

I told her it was okay; we could do both.

"Well, I wanted you to get some rest while you were here."

I said, "I can rest Sunday and Monday before I fly out on Tuesday." I looked at her because she still had this worried look on her face. I told her, "I'm sure."

The next morning, we got up and ate breakfast, fed Mia and Bear, and we were off to hunt down some stone for the exterior walls of the house. As I was driving, Jess was trying to explain the stone that was up in her head to me so I would have an idea what to look for. She was giving me directions at the same time, my little multitasker. We arrived at the first stone place, and the outside was a little creepy. But the inside was nice, and the lady that helped us was really nice as well. We walked all over this place and could not find the stone that my wife was looking for. We went to the second stone store, and they didn't have it either. I told my wife as we were driving to the third store, "Maybe this stone isn't in El Paso."

She said, "I am starting to think the same thing."

I told her, "We have one store left, and hopefully they will have it."

Now this whole time my wife was explaining how this stone looked to me for the past two or three hours. I think she burned it into my subconscious. When I opened the door for her to go into the store, she went straight to the counter. I walked in behind her, and something said to me, "Look to your right." I looked to my right, and there it was, the stone that my wife had implanted into my subconscious. I yelled, "I found it, Jess!" She ran from the counter as the guy was giving her his card. She said, "You found it!" I told her we found it together. We gathered all the pricing information on the stone, and we were out the door.

We were on a good pace and could get to the appliance builder warehouse and just take our time. We pulled up, and my wife jumped out of the car first. Now, my wife never beats me out of the car unless she was super excited, which she was, because she was already around the corner of the building before I closed my door. Normally, she would wait for me to come around the car, not this time. She was on a mission. Me, I was running on fumes by this time because I was out in the sun all week, working, before I flew in to El Paso. But I was determined to keep up with her in the store, and the coolness of the AC in the building helped with that.

Once I caught up with her, I told her it was like a magnet just pulled her in the store as soon as she stepped out of the car. She said, "I'm sorry, I'm just overly excited because I have been waiting a long time for this moment to pick out appliances."

I told her it was no problem, and "now let's get down to business." Everyone was walking around, but we didn't know who to ask about the appliances. So we started walking to the back and looking around.

A lady approached us and introduced herself. "Hi, my name is Helen, and how can I help you?" We told her we were getting our first house built. The builder had scheduled us an appointment today to pick out our appliances. Helen said, "Well, congratulations on your new house. I know you guys are very excited." We both nodded our heads yes. She started explaining the different models all the way up to the high subzero appliances.

When she stopped moving, she stopped right in front of this large refrigerator-freezer combo, and it was stainless steel. I almost walked up to it and gave it a big hug as to say, "There you are, nice to meet you, you want to go home with us today?" But I soon woke up from that dream when my wife asked how much was it. Helen said it was $12,000. I told both of them, "You do realize you can walk right down to the Fiat dealership and buy one of those little cars off their lot for that much, right?"

Helen looked at me and said, "Yep."

My wife said, "Oh no, we're not getting this because we have a budget to stick to."

Helen said, "You guys are welcome to continue looking around. If you find anything, my office is right over there." She pointed to the back of the building.

Jess and I walked around, still looking. She said, "If we could find that same style refrigerator-freezer combo in a less expensive brand, we're getting it today."

I was like, "Okay, let's do this because they have to have something in this store just like it but a different brand."

We made our way to the other side of the front of the store. We were slowly making our way to the back, where Helen's office was located, when my wife let out this big scream in the store, "Look, oh my gosh, look!" Helen came out of her office because she heard my wife. Jess was standing in front of a refrigerator-freezer combo that was stainless steel made by a different manufacturer. She quickly asked Helen how much it was. Helen went back to her office to locate the price.

While she was gone, Jess asked me, "Do you see anyone around?" I looked around because I could see the entire side of the store. I turned and told her there was no one around. Then she hugged the refrigerator. While she was hugging the refrigerator, this lady and her kid came from out of nowhere and looked at my wife, smiling. My wife looked at them and smiled back as she was still hugging the refrigerator. I told her to stop hugging it before Helen saw her.

Jess let go of the refrigerator just as Helen was returning with the price. Helen said the refrigerator was $5,700. My wife and I couldn't believe it. We asked, "Are you sure that is the right price?" Helen said she checked it twice to make sure. Jess pulled out her paperwork and her calculator and started doing her math thing. She looked up and said, "We will take it. We have an allowance on our appliances from the builder, and the refrigerator the builder is offering is $3,300, so only thing we pay is the difference, which is $2,400. Baby we got it … our refrigerator."

Helen called us in her office and told us the company was offering a small rebate on it for $400. "So the new total you will owe is—"

Before Helen could get it out, my wife said, "Just $2,000, even better." Jess and I both didn't realize what had just happened. I mean, really, it all happened so fast.

Before we went to bed that night, my wife went into her vision box and started pulling out things that had manifested for her. At the very bottom of the box was a picture of the refrigerator-freezer combo. She held it for a while, stared at it for a minute or two, before she said, "Look at this, baby." I was blown away because like her, I had forgotten it was in there. We fell asleep talking about how amazing that day was, finding everything like that. Jess said, "Thank you for today, because I knew you were tired."

I told her, "I was a little tired when we got to the appliance store, but once I got into the cool AC, I was good, plus the excitement kept me going as well."

Jess said, "You are resting the rest of the time you're home, okay?"

I said, "Will do."

Tuesday morning rolled around. It wasn't so bad getting dropped off at the airport. I felt like we had accomplished so much that past weekend with our house and everything. My wife was in her happy place with everything that was going on with our house and her job. My son was doing good with his job as well. Mia and Bear were always happy as long as you were giving them food and wrestling with them.

Well, soon after I came back home that last time, the house was complete, and Jess had moved in with the help of the moving company. Franki and some of her Realtor friends helped Jess with the move and garage sale as well. See, I told you Franki was an awesome Realtor, and we didn't even ask for her help. She volunteered. Jess was so grateful to have their help.

Three or four weeks had passed when I came back to El Paso to our new home. That first morning I woke up to the smell of breakfast. I was staring at the design on the ceiling and at the fireplace at the foot of the bed. Thinking to myself, *Wow, it wasn't a dream, this is all real.* I jumped up out of bed, got dressed, went in the bathroom, and started playing with all the light switches like a little kid. I went into the kitchen and gave my wife a big hug and a kiss.

She said to me, "Did you go into the bathroom yet and check everything out?" I told her I was playing with the light switches like a little kid. She said, "There is another surprise in the bathroom for you."

I said, "Are you serious, and you were able to keep it a surprise this long?"

"I almost told you a couple of times. Come with me."

We walked to the master bedroom, and Jess told me to look at the bathtub handles. I said, "Okay, what am I looking at?"

She said, "How many do you see?"

I said, "I see three, so what? Wait a minute ... what are three handles doing here? Did the builder screw up on this?"

Jess was like, "No ... turn the big handle, it's your surprise, baby."

I turned the big handle, and water poured from the ceiling. I was so surprised! I told my wife, "This is what I saw on one of the house channel shows! Wow, and you remember me saying something about this months ago before we even started building the house?"

Jess said, "Yes, I did, and I thought it would make a great surprise for you." I told her it was a great surprise and that I loved it, even though I didn't like surprises.

We then walked back into the kitchen to finish cooking breakfast. Jess walked over to the super large refrigerator and stood in the door for at least two or three minutes. I didn't see her head moving around, scanning for something like she normally would. I asked her if she was okay. She closed the refrigerator and turned with tears running down her face. I walked over to her and hugged her. "Are you okay?" She said she was just so happy to have the house and happy that she was healthy and so very grateful for me for being by her side through everything. I told her that I loved her with all my big heart and that I was so proud of her to be able to overcome so much these past couple of years. We just continued to hug each other.

I am a very grateful husband, best friend, and caregiver.

A message from my wife:

When we wrote this book, we left out a lot of the medical technicalities on purpose. We are not doctors. Our intention is to show you that you can face a traumatic experience head-on and come out okay on the other side. You can still laugh and have fun living without torturing yourself in your mind with all the bad stuff. I think that's what got me in this situation in the first place.

My mom was having a hard time finding the good things she still had in her life, the things she could have still been grateful for. I truly believe that is what brought on her cancer. She worried about everything nonstop and got to the point of constant depression. It was like she fell into this deep hole of despair in her mind and couldn't find her way out. Then one day, she just gave up completely, and that was the end of her life here on earth.

I started replaying things in my mind. Did I do something wrong? Was it my fault she was so depressed? I remembered how upset she got when I went off to college. She was even more upset when Anthony and I moved across the country. Every time we moved, she seemed to get more upset. Could I have done things differently, would it even have made a difference? This went on for a couple weeks.

Then I got diagnosed with stage 4. I was thinking, "What happened to stage 1, 2, and 3?" I knew I had to change my mind-set immediately. I was determined not to give up, no matter what the doctors told me. I remember one doctor saying something about a fifty-fifty chance. I dismissed that right away. I was never giving up! They could have told me seventy-thirty—NEVER GIVING UP!

My first oncologist told me that I didn't have to change my diet. I could eat whatever I wanted. Even though there is a ton of research showing sugar feeds cancer, she said nothing about it. I am glad that I didn't just go on what my doctors advised. Anthony and I took it upon ourselves to do our own research. I knew somewhere inside me that the right nutrition could help. Even if it was just to help cope with the effects of chemo, why not just do a little digging and find out? couldn't hurt anything. Never give up.

That was when we made our lifestyle change. No more refined sugars, only honey and agave in moderation to sweeten things. No more wheat or dairy. No candy, sweets, desserts, sugary drinks. No fast food. Work out more. It's a lifestyle change. It's simple, not necessarily easy. But I did it because I chose life over everything else. Never give up.

People ask me all the time if I want some of their birthday cake or the cookies they made over the weekend. The answer is always "No, thank you" with a smile. At work, I am surrounded by it. Almost every one of my coworkers has at least one bowl full of candy on their desk. Sometimes it just makes me sick to see it. How do they not know it is hurting them on the inside, all for a tiny moment of "pleasure"? Never give up.

There are not enough words to describe how amazing my husband is. It took a lot of courage for him to tell you our story. It took a lot of courage for him to stay by my side through this incredible journey. It took a lot of courage for him to not give up on me and walk out the door. My son, Anthony Jr., has the same courage. He never left either. Never give up.

My entire being overflows with gratitude for my husband, his strength and courage. I make it a point to tell him every day that I am grateful for him. I am grateful for every single day I have here on earth. I am grateful for this journey, which may sound weird, but it has shown us what we are capable of. This journey has shown us how strong we can be. That strength lies within you. Never give up.

Anthony made a choice to stay with me. I made a choice to live. I have a purpose for being here, and so do you. All you have to do is make your choice. Never give up.

About the Author

The author was born in Texarkana, Texas, and lived there until he joined the Army after high school. He served one tour and then decided to attend college, where he met his wife, Jessica. He played football for many years, retiring from the sport after three seasons in the Arena Football League.

Now, he enjoys spending as much time as possible with his wife, son, and two bulldogs, Bear and Mia. He likes working out, lifting weights, riding bike, playing tennis, and going for walks with his beautiful wife.

He hopes their story brings you inspiration, laughter, and strength to make it through life's unexpected speed bumps.